PLACEBO

PLACEBO

The Belief Effect

Dylan Evans

HarperCollins*Publishers*

HarperCollins*Publishers*
77–85 Fulham Palace Road,
Hammersmith, London W6 8JB

The HarperCollins website address is
www.**fire**and**water**.co.uk

Published by HarperCollins*Publishers* 2003
Copyright © Dylan Evans 2003

The author asserts the moral right to
be identified as the author of this work

A catalogue record for this book
is available from the British Library

ISBN 0 00 712612 3

Set in PostScript Monotype Bembo by
Rowland Phototypesetting Limited
Bury St Edmunds, Suffolk

Printed and bound in Great Britain by
Clays Ltd, St Ives plc

CONTENTS

ACKNOWLEDGEMENTS

Thanks are due to my editor at HarperCollins, Richard Johnson, and my agent, Louise Greenberg, for their editorial assistance and publishing expertise. The following people all read various bits and pieces of the book and gave me many useful suggestions for improvement: Ellie Barnes, Caroline Bresson, Romay Garcia, Jonathan Glover, Wilson Harvey, Nicholas Humphrey, Nick Shea and Stephen Senn. Robert Lacey provided excellent copy-editing.

Last but not least, this book would simply not have been possible without the help of Emma Marshall. In addition to providing encouragement throughout, Emma also read and commented on many versions of the manuscript, and spent many long hours in libraries collecting the source material on which this book is based. This book is dedicated to her.

PREFACE

'What we are today comes from our thoughts of yesterday, and our present thoughts build our life of tomorrow: our life is the creation of our mind.'[1] The opening words of the *Dhammapada*, one of the most revered Buddhist scriptures, articulate an ancient and pervasive idea – the mind is all-powerful, and no element of physical reality is beyond its reach. In the West, too, the supremacy of mind over matter is championed by religious movements old and new. Christians and New Age devotees alike agree that the blind can be made to see, and invalids be made to walk, by the power of faith alone.

Science tells a rather different story. The power of the mind, it says, is strictly limited. Every effect it has on the world beyond the body must pass through the prosaic and puny conduit of muscle-power. The victim of total paralysis is completely impotent, his mind entombed, as the medical term – 'locked-in syndrome' – makes painfully clear. Except for the single flutter of an eyelid, which may be the only muscle to remain under voluntary control, the paralytic has no way of influencing the world around him.

But what of the world within? Even science recognises that the brain governs more than the muscles. The discovery, in the 1980s, of the rich supply of nerves linking the brain with the immune system led to the rise of a new branch of medical research known as psychoneuroimmunology (PNI). Advances in PNI have raised hopes that the powers of the mind may not be quite as impoverished as most scientists have thought. Telekinesis and extra-sensory perception may be forever alien to the scientific worldview, but perhaps scientists need not be so pessimistic when it comes to the mind's capacity to influence events within one's own body. Walking on water may be out of the question, but maybe – just maybe – science might discover that disease can be cured by thought alone. Will science, having exposed so many magical powers as mere fantasies, at least allow this one to stand? The heavens have been lost to Copernicus, and creation has been vanquished by Darwin. But the soul, perhaps, still lurks in the healing power of the mind.

That phrase – 'the healing power of the mind' – could cover a multitude of sins. Many sorts of phenomena might fall under its umbrella. Relaxation, for example, lowers blood pressure and may reduce the risk of coronary heart disease. There is nothing particularly magical about that, however. This book is about something much stranger – the possibility of a direct effect of belief on the body, an effect that is not achieved by means of any muscle, not even by the muscles that control our breathing.

Some of the apparent strangeness of the belief effect is almost certainly due to the ethereal images that are still conjured up in many people's imaginations by the term 'mind'. Despite the amazing scientific advances that have transformed our understanding of the brain during the past few decades, it is still common to find people speaking about the mind as if it were something completely separate from the body. While this manner of speaking is thousands of years old, it was most influentially given expression almost four centuries ago by the French philosopher René Descartes (1596–1650). Descartes argued that minds and bodies were composed of completely different kinds of substance – one spiritual in nature, the other material. Given this starting point, it is hard indeed to see how minds can affect bodies, or how bodies can affect minds. And yet they clearly do affect each other. Before I typed this sentence out on the keyboard of my computer, the words formed in my mind; when my fingers then struck the keys, their movement was yet another mundane example of the power of mind over matter. Likewise, if my mood improves after sipping a glass of wine, this is an equally familiar case of the body affecting the mind.

Descartes proposed a rather bizarre theory to explain how the mind and the body were able to communicate with one another. He claimed that a tiny structure in the brain known as the pineal gland acted as a kind of spiritual telephone, enabling messages to be sent back and forth between the ethereal mind and the material body. If that was really the case, of course, we would be able to turn people into mindless zombies simply by removing their pineal glands. Unfortunately for Descartes' theory, however, people whose pineal glands are destroyed do not suddenly turn into zombies. In the centuries since Descartes, we have learned enough about the brain to know that the mind cannot be tied down to any particular part, such as the pineal gland. This is not because the mind uses lots of other regions of the brain to communicate with the body – it is because the mind is simply another name for the activity of the brain.

We know now that the processes of thinking and wishing that Descartes ascribed to the ethereal, invisible mind are, in fact, complex patterns of electro-chemical activity that swirl around in the lump of fatty tissue we call the brain. There is no need for any spiritual telephone to link the brain to the mind, because 'the mind' is just another name for what the brain does. This 'astonishing hypothesis' – as Nobel Prize-winner Francis Crick has called it – removes at one fell swoop a lot of the apparent mystery of that confusing phrase 'the mind–body problem'. What is the problem, when the mind is simply the activity of one part of the body? The mystery turns out to be an artefact of our confused ways of speaking, such as our tendency to persist in talking about 'mind over matter', as if the mind were not itself a material process. If there is any problem at all, it is that of understanding how one part of the body – the brain – communicates with the rest.

★   ★   ★

In the early days of scientific psychology, at the end of the nineteenth century, there was a very simple picture of how the brain and the body communicated. First, certain bits of the body – the sensory organs, such as the eyes and ears – provided information to the brain via the sensory nerves. Then, after the brain had worked out what to do on the basis of this information, it passed the command on to the muscles by means of motor neurons. As our understanding of physiology and anatomy increased, however, it became clear that the situation was far more complex. For a start, the 'five senses' of vision, hearing, taste, touch and smell turned out to be much less monolithic than was previously thought. Touch, for example, is not a single process, but a combination of many different ones; various kinds of receptors in the skin are designed to detect different types of stimuli, such as heat, pressure and chemicals. Also, it has become clear that the brain does not just receive information from the outside world but also from a rich array of sensory nerves that permeate our internal organs. The information they convey to the brain is vital in co-ordinating many physiological processes, even though this information rarely becomes the object of conscious attention.

Still more exciting has been the discovery that some information about the internal state of the body is conveyed to the brain not via sensory nerves, but via chemicals in the bloodstream. Many of these molecular messengers are secreted by white blood cells, whose main role is to help the body fight infection. This has led some biologists to argue that the immune system is itself a kind of sensory organ.[2] Just as the eyes detect visual information about the outside world, so the various components of the immune system are continually monitoring the inside of our bodies for signs of infection, and alerting the brain when they discover them.

The discovery that we possess internal senses as well as external ones is paralleled by the finding that the motor neurons are not the only means by which the brain sends its messages back to the rest of the body. Besides telling the muscles how to move, the brain can also instruct immune cells to change their activity. Certain parts of the brain are designed to secrete certain chemicals back into the bloodstream, and some of these chemical messengers are picked up by white blood cells, which can alter their behaviour accordingly. As we learn more about the ways in which the brain communicates with the rest of the body, it is becoming clear that mental processes need not start with external perception and end in external movement. Some can originate and terminate in events deep inside the body.

It is to this process of internal communication between the brain and the body that I refer when I speak about the healing power of the mind, not to any miraculous Cartesian spiritual telephone. Yet my sense of wonder is undiminished. In my opinion, the scientific discoveries that have allowed us to glimpse the mechanisms that underlie the complex interactions between our beliefs and our health are even more fascinating than the more mystical talk about 'energies' and 'auras' that titillates some. And the scientific story does have one notable advantage that the mystical ones lack – it is based on fact rather than fiction.

Unfashionable as it may be to say so at a time of growing interest in alternative medicine and faith healing, the power of the mind to heal the body is entirely dependent on the various physical mechanisms just described. If there is no chemical messenger to act as a go-between, the brain is powerless to alter the action of the immune system. And even when such molecules do exist, they cannot endow the immune system with supernatural powers. All they can do is tell the immune system to behave in one way rather than another. If something is beyond the power of the immune system altogether, no amount of chemical messengers secreted by the brain will change this.

Rather than attempting to cover every conceivable avenue by which the mind might heal the body, from hypnosis to relaxation, I have chosen to focus on one particular phenomenon – the placebo response. The advantage of focusing on this process, rather than any other, is that science has something to say about it. While it is certainly possible that there are other processes that allow the mind to heal the body, next to nothing is known about them. This is not to say that scientists have a complete picture of the placebo response – far from it, in fact. But there is just about enough scientific research to enable some reasonably solid hypotheses to be developed and tested. And more data is accumulating, as more funds are increasingly devoted to elucidating the mechanisms that underlie the placebo response.

As we shall see in Chapter One, inert substances such as bread pills and salt water have long been used by doctors as sops to desperate patients. In the twentieth century, however, medical researchers began to suspect that placebos such as these might actually have real therapeutic effects. By the 1950s, it had become established medical wisdom that placebos could help to alleviate virtually any disease. More recently, researchers have unearthed significant flaws in this early research, leading some to doubt the very existence of the placebo response. Chapter Two sifts through the evidence to put together a picture of what placebos really can and can't do. The interesting question is not whether placebos can alleviate medical problems – they can – but *which* medical problems they affect.

The list of medical conditions that respond to placebos is a rather odd one, without apparent rhyme or reason. Yet, as Chapter Three argues, there is in fact a single biological mechanism that is common to them all. If this mechanism is *activated* in all these medical conditions, it follows that placebos might work by turning this mechanism off. I may be wrong, and the placebo response may involve other mechanisms. If so, some of the predictions that follow from the model put forward here will not stand up to empirical test. That strikes me as a virtue rather than a disadvantage. Good theories, as the philosopher of science Karl Popper never tired of repeating, must be falsifiable. The bolder the conjectures, the more chances of being shown to be wrong, the better the theory. The theory put forward here is consistent with most, if not all, the data we currently have about the placebo response. But these are early days, and it is perfectly possible that scientists may discover further data that prove the theory wrong.

Such an event would not invalidate the whole book. Most of the arguments in its second half would still hold up even if the theory advanced in Chapter Three turns out to be wrong. Whatever the physiological details may be, for example, the important thing about placebos is that they cause their bodily effects indirectly, by means of causing some change in the mind. Chapter Four looks at the psychological element in the placebo response, the key mental event that triggers the physiological processes involved. I argue that this mental event is the formation of a belief – the belief that one has just received an effective medical treatment. Placebos are treatments that only work if you believe in them.

Chapter Five puts the physiological and psychological mechanisms in an evolutionary context. How and why did humans evolve in such a way that their minds can trick their bodies into healing themselves? When did this capacity first appear? Chapter Six examines the so-called 'nocebo effect' – the power of placebos to harm as well as to heal – and argues that this crude dichotomy into good and bad seriously misrepresents the complexity of the biological details. Since many symptoms turn out to be defence mechanisms activated by the body itself, it is much harder than one might think to decide whether or not a physiological process is pathological or beneficial.

Chapters Seven and Eight take a hard look at alternative medicine and psychotherapy, and ask whether or not these popular approaches to healing are really anything more than placebos. The question is especially important at a time when consumer demand for these products is high. Should we believe the hype surrounding acupuncture and homeopathy, or is the emperor naked?

Finally, Chapter Nine looks at the ethical questions raised by the use of placebos. To use a placebo knowingly, whether in medical practice or in clinical trials, it seems that doctors must deceive their patients. Can such deception ever be justified, or do doctors have an absolute duty to tell their patients the truth? And how do the emerging scientific discoveries discussed earlier in the book throw new light on this ancient dilemma?

That concludes the rough sketch of the terrain; now begins the journey.

Dylan Evans
Fairford
July 2002

Chapter 1

PLACEBOS ON TRIAL

In the closing years of World War II, while the Allies were fighting to liberate Europe from German occupation, morphine was in great demand at the military field hospitals. When casualties were particularly heavy, demand would outstrip supply and operations had to be performed without analgesia. On one such occasion, Henry Beecher, an American anaesthetist, was preparing to treat a soldier with terrible injuries. He was worried; without morphine, not only would the operation be extremely painful – it might even induce a fatal cardiovascular shock. But then something very strange happened, something that was profoundly to alter Beecher's view of medicine for the rest of his life. In desperation, one of the nursing staff injected the patient with a harmless solution of saline. To Beecher's surprise, the patient settled down immediately, just as if he had been given morphine. Not only did the soldier seem to feel very little pain during the subsequent operation, but the full-blown shock did not develop either.[1] Salt water, it seemed, could be just as effective as one of the most powerful painkillers in the medical arsenal. In the following months, when supplies of morphine again ran low, Beecher repeated the trick. It worked. Beecher returned to America after the war convinced of the power of placebos, and gathered around him at Harvard a group of colleagues to study the phenomenon.

Around the same time, others were also beginning to take an interest in the placebo response. Harry Gold, at Cornell

1

University, had been working on the topic independently since before the war. His work on angina had convinced him, like Beecher, that placebos could exert powerful therapeutic effects. In 1946, Gold led a discussion about the use of placebos in therapy at a conference at Cornell.[2] Soon after, Beecher's team at Harvard embarked on a series of studies comparing the effectiveness of analgesics with that of placebos. By 1955 interest in the placebo response had grown to such an extent that one of Beecher's colleagues, Louis Lasagna, was even invited to write about the topic in *Scientific American*.[3]

The scientific interest in placebos was new. Although doctors had been quietly using sugar pills and water injections as sops to placate desperate patients for many years before Beecher started running his studies, few regarded the practice as worthy of serious research. Quite the contrary; physicians often felt rather uneasy about the whole business. It smacked of quackery and fraud. Doctors justified the practice of handing out placebos on the grounds that it could do no harm, but did not think for a moment that it actually helped patients to get better. An article in the *Lancet* in 1954 summed up this old-fashioned view of the placebo as 'a means of reinforcing a patient's confidences in his recovery, when the diagnosis is undoubted and no more effective treatment is possible'. The article went on to note that 'for some unintelligent or inadequate patients life is made easier by a bottle of medicine to comfort their ego; that to refuse a placebo to a dying incurable patient may simply be cruel; and that to decline to humour an elderly "chronic" brought up on the bottle is hardly within the bounds of possibility'.[4]

This view of the placebo as a 'humble humbug', as the *Lancet* article was so aptly titled, echoes the etymology of the term. *Placebo* is Latin for 'I will please'. In the Latin translation of the Bible that was used throughout the Middle Ages, the word occurs as part of Psalm 116 – the part that was used in the Catholic vespers for the dead. People who wanted these prayers sung for their recently-deceased loved ones would be charged exorbitant fees by the priests and friars who performed the sacred rites. The priests, we may suppose, did not share the same sense of loss as those in mourning, and so the expression *placebo* came to stand as a pejorative shorthand for any form of words that was insincere but perhaps consoling nonetheless. This is the sense in which Chaucer used the term in the fourteenth century, when he wrote that 'flatterers are the devil's chaterlaines for ever singing placebo'. Over two hundred years later, Francis Bacon also had flatterers in mind when he advised kings to beware of their advisers:

> A king, when he presides in counsel, let him beware how he opens his own inclination too much, in that which he propoundeth; for else counsellors will but take the wind of him, and instead of giving free counsel, sing him a song of placebo.

In the eighteenth century, *placebo* entered the medical lexicon as a term for fake remedies. When the physician thought nothing was wrong with a patient, he might give him a bread pill or some other innocuous substance just to keep him happy. This way, the patient would at least be spared the danger of taking a real treatment when nothing was wrong with him. In 1807, the American President Thomas Jefferson wrote in his diary that one of the most successful physicians he had ever known had assured him that 'he used more bread pills, drops of coloured water and powders of hickory ash than all other medicines put together'. Jefferson added that he considered this practice 'a pious fraud' – a phrase which nicely captures both aspects of the original use of the term *placebo*. Just like a prayer for the dead sung by monks who never knew the deceased, a bread pill was both deceptive and consoling, a white lie to cover up a nasty fact.

All this changed after World War II. The studies conducted by Beecher, Gold, Lasagna and other elite medical researchers revolutionised the way doctors thought about placebos. By the mid-1950s, the medical profession was beginning to think that handing out placebos might not be such a fraudulent practice after all. Experiments had shown that inactive substances could induce similar effects to those of caffeine and alcohol when people were fooled into thinking that the innocuous liquids they were given contained coffee or wine. Perhaps equally powerful effects could be produced by the bread pills given out by physicians. Perhaps placebos could really heal people.

PLACEBOS BECOME RESPECTABLE

In 1955, Beecher summed up the new view of placebos in an influential article published in the *Journal of the American Medical Association*.[5] Entitled 'The Powerful Placebo', the article claimed that placebos could 'produce gross physical change', including 'objective changes at the end organ which may exceed those attributable to potent pharmacological action'. Placebos, in other words, had real effects on real bodies. No longer were sugar pills to be dismissed as a harmless but ineffectual sop given to please hypochondriacs and desperate people. The placebo effect was born.

Beecher's article has been enormously influential. Fifty years after publication, it is still regularly cited in almost every scientific paper on the placebo effect, and even those that do not cite it directly usually repeat its claims without acknowledgement, or refer to papers that do cite it. It is unlikely, however, that all of those who refer to it have bothered to read it; if they had done, they might not be quite so enthusiastic. For one thing, the range of conditions that Beecher claims can be affected by placebos is not very extensive. Most of the studies he reports concern the effects of placebos on various forms of pain – postoperative pain, pain from angina and headache. The only other medical problems mentioned are cough, common cold, seasickness and anxiety, and for each of these Beecher mentions only one study. More importantly, none of the studies he refers to provides any real evidence at all for the existence of a placebo effect.

The reason why these early studies provide no evidence of

a placebo effect is that, with one exception, all failed to include a control group who received no treatment. In any group of people suffering from a particular condition, some will get better without any medical help. To provide convincing evidence of a placebo effect, you would have to show that those receiving the placebo did significantly better than those who received no treatment at all. Yet almost all the studies cited by Beecher merely show that some of those who received a placebo – a third, on average – felt better afterwards. Without a no-treatment control group to compare it with, this figure is meaningless. The improvement shown by those who received the placebo might well have occurred anyway, even if they had received no placebo. The one study that did include a no-treatment group found no difference between it and the placebo group.

The authors of the original studies did not think they had found any evidence of placebo effects. A few of them even said so explicitly. They realised that the improvement shown by those receiving placebos could easily be accounted for by the natural course of the disease (spontaneous remission, random fluctuation of symptoms and so on) and various other factors such as additional treatments. In one of the studies, for example, 35 per cent of the patients with mild colds felt better within two days of taking a placebo (or six days after the start of their cold). The authors of the study pointed out that many patients with a mild cold get better within six days even if they receive no medical treatment at all. Beecher, however, ignored this remark, and attributed all the improvement shown by these patients to the fact that they had taken a placebo.

Besides spontaneous remission, other factors also play a part in the improvement shown by patients receiving placebos. In one study cited by Beecher, for example, patients with a variety of conditions were treated for anxiety and tension. After four months, during which they were given two-week courses of an anti-anxiety drug called mephensin and placebo alternately, between 20 and 30 per cent of them improved. However, another 10–20 per cent of patients deteriorated. The authors of the study subtracted the deterioration rate from the improvement rate and reported, correctly, a net improvement of around 10 per cent. Considering the rather long observation period of sixteen weeks, this seems quite a low figure, especially when one considers that the patients had taken an active drug for eight of the sixteen weeks. Some of them may also have received other medical support outside the context of the study. Yet Beecher failed to take the deterioration rate into account, and claimed that the study showed a placebo effect of 30 per cent.

In fact, Beecher misquoted ten of the fifteen trials he cited – including one which he had co-authored himself.[6] His cavalier attitude in reporting these studies is paradoxical, since his underlying objective in marshalling evidence for the placebo effect was to persuade medical researchers to be more rigorous in their approach to evaluating new treatments. Before World War II, the evaluation of new therapies was largely determined by the personal judgement of distinguished doctors. Beecher was a leading figure in the movement to reform this long tradition. Along with Gold and others, he argued vigorously that medical treatments could best be tested by a new method: the randomised, placebo-controlled clinical trial.

THE LONG BIRTH OF THE CLINICAL TRIAL

As to different methods of treatment, it is possible for us to assure ourselves of the superiority of one or another . . . by enquiring if the greater number of individuals have been cured by one means than another. Here it is necessary to count. And it is, in great part at least, because hitherto this method has not at all, or rarely been employed, that the science of therapeutics is so uncertain.
PIERRE LOUIS, *Essay on Clinical Instruction* (1834)

In some ways, the clinical trial was not new. Something very similar is described in as venerable a text as the Old Testament. The first chapter of the Book of Daniel describes how Nebu-

chadnezzar, King of Babylon, offered his own food to some of
the most noble Israelites he had taken prisoner after capturing
the city of Jerusalem. Daniel refused to eat the foreign food,
since it did not conform to the Jewish dietary laws. Nebuchad-
nezzar's chief eunuch was sympathetic, but warned Daniel that
his own head would be in danger if the King saw him looking
thinner in the face than the other Israelites. At this, Daniel
turned to the guard and made a request: 'Please allow your
servants a ten-day trial, during which we are given only veg-
etables to eat and water to drink. You can then compare our
looks with those of the boys who eat the King's food.' The
guard agreed, and after ten days Daniel, and the friends who
had accompanied him on his vegetarian diet, looked in better
shape than those who had eaten at the royal table. This is not
exactly a clinical trial – for one thing, it concerns a dietary
regime rather than a medical treatment – but the basic idea of
comparing an experimental group with a control group is there.

Historians have unearthed various other ancient progenitors
of the modern clinical trial. In the thirteenth century, the King
of Sicily, Frederick II (1272–1337), is reported to have studied
the effects of exercise on digestion by giving identical meals to
two knights and then sending one out hunting while ordering
the other to bed. After several hours, he killed both and examined the contents of their alimentary canals; digestion had,
apparently, proceeded further in the stomach of the sleeping
knight.[7] A century later, Petrarch reported, in a letter to Boccac-
cio, a remark by a fellow physician that explicitly recommended
experimental studies of therapeutic methods by comparative
means.[8] But, like the story of Daniel, these early gestures toward
comparative studies lack one of the most distinctive features of
the modern clinical trial – a formal mathematical treatment.
This had to wait until the birth of statistics in the seventeenth
century.

Some philosophers and historians of science have argued that
the development of statistics and probability theory in the eighteenth and nineteenth centuries constituted a revolution no less

dramatic and influential than the 'scientific revolution' of the seventeenth century.[9] In reality the so-called 'probabilistic revolution' was a pretty slow affair, more akin to the stately orbit of a celestial body than to a political upheaval. Its impact on medical research was positively sluggish. Statistical methods were not explicitly used to investigate a therapeutic intervention until the 1720s, when the French physician James Jurin showed that smallpox inoculation was a safe procedure by comparing the mortality of inoculated people with the death rates of those with natural smallpox. Even then, the new methods did not meet with much respect; Jurin's findings were ignored by his colleagues, and smallpox inoculation remained illegal in France until 1769.

A hundred years later, the same mistrust of statistical methods led Viennese physicians to reject the recommendations of Ignaz Semmelweis on the need for better hygiene by doctors. In 1847 Semmelweis noticed that there were marked differences between the death rates on two wards in the obstetric hospital in Vienna. Mortality was much higher on the ward run by physicians and medical students than on the ward run by student midwives. Moreover, the difference between the two wards had only begun in 1841, when courses in pathology were included in medical training. Semmelweis guessed that physicians and students were coming to the obstetric ward with particles of corpses from the dissection room still clinging to their fingers. He made them wash more thoroughly with chlorinated lime (which, by luck, just happened to be a disinfectant), and the death rate on the medical ward immediately returned to the same level as on that run by the midwives. Despite this startling evidence, the antiseptic measures proposed by Semmelweis were not embraced by his colleagues for several decades, by which time Semmelweis had, quite understandably, gone insane.

British doctors were, in general, more accepting of statistical research than were their colleagues on the Continent. In the eighteenth century, a few physicians on board British naval vessels employed comparative methods to study the effects of various treatments for scurvy and fever. John Lind noted that sailors on his ship who had scurvy recovered when given citrus fruits, and the navy responded by issuing lemons (and later limes) to all sailors – which is, of course, the origin of the epithet 'limey'. But the British were not so open-minded with all such statistical research. In the late 1860s, Joseph Lister published a series of articles showing that the use of antiseptics at the Glasgow Royal Infirmary had reduced the mortality from amputations, but his findings were not universally accepted by the British medical establishment until the end of the century.

By the first half of the twentieth century, there was a growing acceptance of comparative methods in medical research among doctors in Europe and America, but even then it was a slow process. The term 'clinical trial' does not appear in the medical literature until the early 1930s, and when Linford Rees presented the results of a trial comparing electro-convulsive therapy (ECT) with insulin coma therapy to a meeting of the Royal Medico-Psychological Association in 1949, his research methodology caused as much of a stir as his results.[10] Very few of the psychiatrists at that meeting could have guessed that, within half a century, the randomised clinical trial would have become the standard tool for medical research.

THE PLACEBO CONTROL

The pre-twentieth-century progenitors of the clinical trial established the basic principle of comparing various groups of patients undergoing different treatment regimes. The twentieth century added two more refinements: randomisation and the placebo control. Randomisation simply means that patients are assigned to the various groups on a random basis. The placebo control means that the control group is treated with a fake version of the experimental therapy – one which, ideally, should be identical in every way to the treatment being tested with the exception of the crucial component. With one or two notable exceptions, the few clinical trials that were carried out before World War II did not include a placebo control group. Rather, they compared one treatment with another, or with no treatment at all. Placebos were used as controls in the studies of effects of substances such as caffeine on healthy volunteers, but the idea of deliberately withholding a treatment believed to be active from someone who was ill and in danger of death was felt by most doctors to be unethical.

Beecher played a major role in persuading doctors that placebo controls were both ethical and scientifically necessary. He countered the ethical objections by arguing that the administration of a placebo was far from 'doing nothing'. If placebos could provide at least half as much relief as a real drug, and often even more, then the patients in the control group would not be that much worse off than those in the experimental arm. Similar considerations were used to support the claim that placebo-controlled studies were the most sound from a scientific point of view. After all, if a therapy was simply shown to be better than no treatment at all, how could doctors be sure that the effect was not due to the placebo response? And if one therapy were compared to another and found to be equally effective, how could scientists be sure that *both* were not placebos? By the end of the 1950s, the work by Beecher, Gold and others had convinced most medical researchers that only by comparing a therapy with a placebo could they discover its specific effect.

Beecher argued that all kinds of treatment, even active drugs and invasive surgery, produced powerful placebo effects in addition to their specific effects. Therefore, to determine the specific effect of a treatment, medical researchers would have to subtract the placebo effect from the total therapeutic effect of the treatment being tested. If they simply compared the experimental treatment with a no-treatment control group, they would overestimate the specific effect by confounding it with the placebo effect. To support this argument, Beecher needed to provide evidence showing that the placebo effect was large enough to worry about. This was the whole point of the 1955 article whose many flaws we have briefly glimpsed. Without misquotation and systematic misrepresentation, the original studies that Beecher cited would not have provided the evidence he needed.

At the time, nobody noticed the flaws in Beecher's article. His evidence was cited again and again in support of the placebo-controlled clinical trial, which continued its rise to dominance. Crucial in this process was the decision in the 1970s by the US Food and Drug Administration (FDA) that new drugs be tested by clinical trials before they could be licensed. As one expert on the history of psychiatry has remarked, the FDA occupies something of a magisterial role in global medicine.[11] It has no legal powers to control the health policies of nations other than the United States, yet its influence is enormous. The decision of the FDA to require new drugs to prove their mettle in randomised, placebo-controlled clinical trials paved the way for similar policies in other countries. During the 1980s, scientific journals followed suit by requiring that claims for the efficacy of new drugs be backed up by evidence from clinical trials. Finally, the 1990s saw the emergence of a movement known as 'evidence-based medicine' whose proponents urged GPs to make use of the evidence from clinical trials in their everyday clinical practice.[12]

A FLAW IN THE METHOD

A physician who tries a remedy and cures his patients, is inclined to believe that the cure is due to his treatment. But the first thing to ask them is whether they have tried doing nothing, i.e. not treating other patients; for how can they otherwise know whether the remedy or nature cured them?

CLAUDE BERNARD, *An Introduction to the Study of Experimental Medicine* (1865)

11

To the proponents of evidence-based medicine, the tortured history of the clinical trial is an epic of an almost biblical nature. Its eventual acceptance, in the late twentieth century, as the gold standard of medical research is the triumph of rational medicine over quackery, dimly foreseen by such early prophets as Jurin, Semmelweis and Lister who were, during their day, lone voices crying in the wilderness.

The truth is not quite so simple. The rise to dominance of the clinical trial has not been an unambiguous victory for rational medicine. Beecher saw it as a way of overcoming centuries of blind appeal to authority and intuition. Ironically, however, the final acceptance of placebo controls owed more to Beecher's own authority and intuition than to proper scientific evidence. Beecher was a respected researcher, so nobody paused to question the accuracy of his 1955 paper. Nobody suspected that he had reshaped the data so that they would support his prior intuitions about the power of the placebo effect.

The result is that, fifty years later, many medical researchers accept without question that placebo effects are ubiquitous and powerful. Take this dramatic passage by two experts on alternative medicine, Dr Robert Buckman and Karl Sabbagh, for example:

> . . . placebos are extraordinary drugs. They seem to have some effect on almost every symptom known to mankind, and work in at least a third of patients (usually) and sometimes in up to 60 per cent. They have no serious side-effects and cannot be given in overdose. In short, they hold the prize for the most adaptable, protean, effective, safe and cheap drugs in the world's pharmacopoeia. Not only that, but they've been around for centuries, so even their pedigree is impeccable.[13]

A respected biologist states that 'placebo medical procedures have proved to be effective against a wide range of medical problems including chronic pain, high blood pressure, angina, depression, schizophrenia and even cancer'.[14] A leading authority on alternative medicine goes even further, claiming that 'the range of susceptible conditions appears to be limitless'.[15]

In fact, almost all the supposed 'demonstrations' of the placebo effect on which these hyperbolic claims are based turn out to embody the same flaws that bedevil Beecher's paper. Whenever people in the placebo arm of a clinical trial get better, they assume that this improvement is due entirely to the placebo, without considering any of the other possible causes – spontaneous remission, natural fluctuation of symptoms, other treatments, and so on. If this kind of sloppy thinking was applied to the testing of real drugs, it would be spotted immediately. When it comes to testing placebos, however, rigour goes out of the window. There seems to be a clear double standard in medical research.

To be consistent, we should apply the same rigorous scientific principles to the study of placebos that we apply to the evaluation of real treatments. No scientist would accept claims advanced on behalf of a new drug without evidence that people who are treated with it are at least more likely to get better than those who remain untreated. It should be no different when it comes to the claims made on behalf of placebos. In other words, to calculate the true placebo effect, the rate of spontaneous remission shown by those receiving no treatment at all must be subtracted from the observed placebo effect. Without a no-treatment arm, there is no way to distinguish the effects of the placebo from the natural course of the disease and various other confounding variables, such as other treatments taken outside the context of the trial.

In fact, no-treatment groups are rarely included in clinical trials today. One survey of the medical literature between 1986 and 1994 found that fewer than 4 per cent of clinical trials and meta-analyses published during that period included both placebo and untreated groups.[16] The result is that, despite half a century of placebo-controlled clinical trials, we have surprisingly little solid data about the extent of the placebo response. The lack of such data has even led a few sceptics to argue that the placebo response does not really exist. They claim that the improvement shown by patients receiving placebos in clinical trials is due entirely to spontaneous remission and random fluctuations in the course of the disease.[17]

This is going too far. Solid evidence in favour of the placebo response is hard to find, but it does exist. Some studies do include no-treatment control groups, and some of these show that patients receiving placebos do better than those who receive nothing. But they are few and far between, and they do not always make sure that the only difference between the placebo group and the no-treatment group is the placebo itself. For example, the patients in the placebo group may receive all sorts of extra attention that those in the no-treatment group do not. As a result, we cannot really be sure that any improvement they may show, compared to the no-treatment group, is due to the placebo rather than to the various other things that they received, but which the no-treatment group did not.

THE LIVES TO COME

Medical progress is based on research which ultimately must rest in part on experimentation involving human subjects.
WORLD MEDICAL ASSOCIATION, *Journal of the American Medical Association* (1964)

There are obvious ethical problems with the idea of using a no-treatment control group. To withhold all medical treatment from a group of patients, simply for the sake of scientific research, seems to flout some of the most basic principles of medical ethics. Similar concerns were raised in the late 1940s and early 1950s when Gold, Beecher and others argued for the need to include placebo control groups in clinical trials. How could doctors justify doing nothing for patients who were clearly in need of help, when active treatments were readily available?

As we have already seen, Beecher answered these objections by claiming that giving patients placebos was far from 'doing nothing'. If placebos were as powerful as he argued, then the patients in the control group would not fare much worse than those in the experimental group. The same cannot be said, of course, for those in a no-treatment group. In that case, doctors do not even give a placebo. This seems much harder to justify.

Actually, there are several considerations that make the inclusion of no-treatment groups in clinical trials less ethically dubious than it may initially appear. First, the term 'no-treatment group' is misleading, since patients in such groups need not be deprived of all medical care. In fact, if we are simply interested in measuring the placebo effect, the ideal situation would be for the 'no-treatment' group to be treated in exactly the same way as the placebo group, with the sole exception of not receiving the placebo. Only then could researchers be confident that any differences between the recovery rates of the two groups were due to the administration of the placebo and not some other factor. So the no-treatment group should, ideally, be visited by the doctor as frequently as the placebo group, be given the same encouragement and support, and so on. It would be more accurate to call this a 'no-placebo' group rather than a 'no-treatment' group.

There is also the possibility that the experimental treatment is not, in fact, effective, in which case those who are not receiving it do not suffer by comparison with those who are. This also applies to the placebo treatment. If the placebo effect really is just a myth, as the critics claim, or if placebos simply do not work for the particular medical condition being examined, then giving patients placebos really is not much better than giving them nothing at all. It may make them feel slightly better, but it would have no effect on their disease. In this case, Beecher's justification for including placebo groups in clinical trials falls apart.

There is another ethical consideration, though, that applies equally to both placebo control groups and no-treatment arms, irrespective of whether the placebo effect is real or not. This is the idea that the needs of current patients should be balanced against those of future generations. Depriving a small group of patients for a short time of all treatment might be defensible if it enabled doctors to make discoveries that would benefit vast numbers of future patients. Such moral calculations are notoriously difficult, and have been used to justify the most appalling crimes. Millions of Soviet citizens, for example, were encouraged to put up with draconian social policies by the officially-sponsored belief that their grandchildren would reap the rewards of their labour. Nevertheless, it is doubtful that immediate needs should always trump those of future generations. To call for the introduction of no-treatment groups in clinical trials is not to put the concerns of the disinterested scientist above those of the caring physician. The ultimate beneficiary of good medical research is the patient, not the researcher.

MIND-BODY MEDICINE

If no-treatment control groups were included in clinical trials in addition to the placebo arm, the path would be open to testing the various claims advanced for and against the existence of the placebo effect. But how could this benefit future generations of patients? Arguably, it could help to answer one of the oldest questions in the history of medicine – how much can mind-power alone help the process of physical healing?

This question goes right back to the origin of Western medicine in ancient Greece, when, in the fifth century BC, Hippocrates and his followers began to reject the supernatural explanations that had dominated previous thinking about health and disease. Instead of blaming sickness on malevolent spirits, Hippocrates argued that all disease could be traced to simple physical problems, such as imbalances in the various liquids or 'humours' that circulated around the body. This rejection of psychological influences on health laid the foundations for the body-centred approach of modern Western medicine. It also sowed the seeds for a fierce debate that continues to this day and which has split medicine in two.

Plato was one of the first to take issue with Hippocrates and his followers. 'This is the great error of our day in the treatment of the human body,' he complained, 'that physicians separate the soul from the body.' It was a mistake, he argued, to treat the body without also attending to the soul. Two thousand years later, the same recriminations are still frequently levelled at Western medicine. The rise of alternative and complementary medicine is simply the latest development in a protracted battle between the idea that recovery from disease is a purely physical process and the view that the mind can play a powerful role in healing.

Unfortunately, the exchanges between the proponents of these two opposed views have usually tended to generate more heat than light. Too often each side has assumed the truth of its own position without providing evidence, as if it were obvious, with the result that the position of the other side can only seem like wilful ignorance driven by a hidden agenda. The believers in alternative medicine accuse orthodox medicine of narrow-mindedness, while the sceptics see the rhetoric of the mind-cure movement as an excuse for all manner of quackery, fraud and deception. There is some truth in both of these criticisms. There have undoubtedly been many exaggerated claims advanced on behalf of faith-healing, and the American magician James Randi has exposed many so-called 'miracle cures' as mere illusions and conjuring tricks. On the other hand, many scientists have been too quick to dismiss the whole area of mind-body medicine without examining the evidence fairly. It is time we stepped back and attempted to apply the same scientific principles to the question of mental healing that we apply to physical therapies. Proper research into the placebo effect offers an excellent place to start. In fact, it might be just what medicine needs to heal itself.

PLACEBOS AND CANCER

The idea that the mind can cure even the most deadly diseases, including cancer, is a popular one. It's certainly a very comforting idea, but is it true? The evidence is mixed. David Spiegel and his colleagues at Stanford University have found that taking part in group psychotherapy can help women with advanced breast cancer to survive longer, but there were no miraculous cures.[18] And the mechanisms which underlie this phenomenon are probably quite different from those involved in the placebo response. Spiegel has argued convincingly that the increase in life expectancy was due mainly to the fact that participating in the group psychotherapy sessions led the women to become involved with each other socially.[19] They started to visit each other's houses, encouraged each other when they had medical problems, and visited each other in hospital. The greater social support in turn encouraged the women to make better use of medical facilities, to co-operate more with doctors, and to make greater effort to look after themselves in general. These behavioural mechanisms are very valuable, but they are a far cry from proving any direct effect of the mind on the healing system.

There is only one case recorded in the medical literature that looks like a case of the placebo response curing cancer. It was reported way back in 1957 by an American psychologist called Bruno Klopfer, and concerns a man whom Klopfer dubbed 'Mr Wright'.[20] Mr Wright had advanced cancer of the lymph nodes (lymphoma), and was expected to die within a few weeks. The various treatments of last resort – radiotherapy and an early chemotherapy agent called nitrogen mustard – could not be used because he was anaemic. While he lay in his bed, awaiting death, Mr Wright heard that a new anti-cancer drug called krebiozen was being tested at the same hospital. He pleaded with his doctor to be given some of the new drug, and his doctor gave him a shot.

Within a few days of the injection, Mr Wright was a changed man. No longer bedridden, he was walking around the ward, chatting happily with the nurses. The huge tumour masses dotted around his body had shrunk from the size of oranges to the size of golf balls. Soon after, he was released from the hospital, apparently free of malignancy.

Two months later the newspapers reported that krebiozen was worthless. Mr Wright's tumours quickly returned, and he was back in hospital. At this point, his doctor did something that would today be forbidden; he lied to him. Suspecting that the cure had all been down to Mr Wright's belief in the drug, the doctor told him that the newspapers were wrong, and that krebiozen was turning out to be a powerful remedy for cancer. The only reason for Mr Wright's relapse, the doctor assured him, was that the dose he had been given came from a batch that had deteriorated somewhat while in the pharmacy. Fortunately for Mr Wright, the doctor went on, a new batch of double-strength krebiozen was due to arrive at the hospital in two days' time. Two days later, the doctor started giving Mr Wright injections – of pure water.

Again the tumours melted away, and Mr Wright lived for a further two months without symptoms. Then another newspaper report appeared, this time announcing the final verdict of the American Medical Association: nationwide tests really had shown krebiozen to be useless. Again, Mr Wright's tumours reappeared, and within a few days he was back at the hospital. Two days after his readmission, he was dead.

This story has been repeated many times in the literature on mind-body medicine, but it remains the only one of its kind. This in itself should make us suspicious, since, as we shall see, single cases can be notoriously misleading. True, the timing of the events is very suggestive. Both recoveries happened very shortly after Mr Wright's beliefs about his prognosis had gone from pessimistic to optimistic, and both relapses occurred within a few days of the reverse change. But coincidences do happen.

To rule out coincidence, we would need to know what would have happened to Mr Wright if he hadn't been treated and consequently become so optimistic. Would he still have got better anyway? Of course, we will never really know for sure. We can't go back in time and observe what would have happened if his doctor had never given him the krebiozen or the water injections. We can, however, make an educated guess, based on what tends to happen to people with similar forms of cancer if they are untreated.

There are many forms of cancer, each with its own typical sequence of events. A few, such as lymphoma, are known to fluctuate spontaneously. In a high proportion of cases, the tumours wax and wane without any treatment at all. The fact that Mr Wright was suffering from lymphoma rather than any other form of cancer means that it is quite possible that his two brief remissions from the disease were simply spontaneous fluctuations, unrelated to the krebiozen or the water injections. The fact that the recoveries occurred just after each treatment could easily have been a coincidence. In fact, since no other similar stories have been recorded, this seems the most likely explanation. Despite what some people may say, there is no evidence that the placebo response can cure cancer.

NO EVIDENCE?

'In my experience' is a phrase that usually introduces a statement of rank prejudice or bias. The information that follows it cannot be checked, nor has it been subjected to any analysis other than some vague tally in the speaker's memory.

MICHAEL CRICHTON, *New England Journal of Medicine* (1971)

To say that there is 'no evidence' that the placebo response can cure cancer might seem too strong. After all, there is the story of Mr Wright. Surely, it might be objected, that has *some* evidential value. Andrew Weil, one of the most famous proponents of alternative approaches to medicine, claims that individual case-histories and personal testimonials should be taken more seriously by medical scientists. He values 'anecdotal evidence' and wonders, with a hint of Freudian suspicion, 'why so many doctors have a hard time with it'.[21]

In fact, the scepticism shown by many doctors today towards claims based on individual case-histories has nothing to do with any emotional unease. If anything, it is statistics that doctors have a hard time with, rather than individual case-histories. Doctors have to learn to override their natural tendencies to be swayed by personal narrative and anecdote, and it is not an easy lesson. It is a vitally important one, though, as the history of medicine has shown, over and over again, that anecdotes are worthless without a proper statistical analysis. Many hundreds of ideas about the origins of disease and claims for surefire remedies have been accepted by doctors on the basis of 'anecdotal evidence', only to be shown, by eventual statistical analysis, to be completely false. Take bloodletting, for example. The technique was first introduced in Egypt around 1000 BC, and then spread to Europe via Greece. For almost three thousand years it was the mainstay of medical practice in the West. Every doctor could testify to its efficacy from his own experience, and tell dozens of anecdotes about how a certain patient got better after being bled. No attempt was made to evaluate bloodletting by statistical methods until the nineteenth century, when the French physician Pierre Louis and others found that it was useless at best, and at worst positively harmful. Only then did doctors finally abandon the ancient technique that had been handed down to them by generations of physicians, all of whom had been convinced it was therapeutic.

As has already been noted, the statistical methods of modern medical research have attracted more than their fair share of critical remarks. These criticisms reveal much about human preferences, but nothing about the value of statistics. Certainly, stories of individual patients and their triumphs over disease grip us in a way that statistics do not. This is what makes the self-help books and the New Age treatises so convincing. These volumes are littered with amazing anecdotes about this person's miraculous recovery from cancer, or that person's amazing triumph over arthritis. Such books are notoriously lacking in statistics. The serious scientific books that *do* contain statistics, on the other hand, leave most of us cold and unconvinced. The personal immediacy of a single human narrative tends to have more impact than the dry numerical objectivity of a mass of statistics.

21

It takes a real effort of will to pay more attention to the statistical information, but this is what we must do if we are to make our decisions on a rational basis rather than by hearsay and rumour. Statistics may be unromantic, but they are a vital remedy for the instinctive human tendency to be persuaded by isolated cases and individual stories. Of course, the statistics need to be interpreted with care, and this requires skill, intelligence and patient attention to mathematical detail. And not even the most sophisticated clinical trial can guarantee truth. It follows from the very nature of statistical research that some clinical trials are bound to generate false conclusions. The doctor and writer James Le Fanu has observed that statistical research 'has been shown to result in the adoption of ineffective treatments in 32 per cent of cases'.[22] The irony of this remark should be clear; we only know that statistical research is flawed because of statistics. There is a more serious point, however, and that is that 'anecdotal evidence' is even less reliable than statistical evidence. Statistics are not infallible, but when it comes to medical research, they are the best tool we have.

THE HIERARCHY OF EVIDENCE

The hard-won lessons about the relative value of anecdotal and statistical evidence have been condensed by medical researchers into a simple formula that is now referred to as the 'hierarchy of evidence'.[23] Individual case-histories and clinical vignettes are quite properly located at the bottom of the ladder. Strictly speaking, then, we should not dismiss such stories altogether, but rather emphasise their limited evidential value. Various statistical methods of research are assigned different grades on the hierarchy of evidence, with randomised controlled trials coming very near the top. The pinnacle of the hierarchy, however, is reserved not for individual clinical trials, but for systematic reviews and meta-analyses. In these research papers, all the clinical trials on a particular topic are hunted down and their results analysed by means of yet more statistical devices.

The prestige attached to meta-analysis, a set of statistical techniques developed in the 1970s, by medical researchers has not met with universal agreement. One epidemiologist, for example, has written that 'meta-analysis begins with scientific studies, usually performed by academics or government agencies, and sometimes incomplete or disputed. The data from the studies are then run through computer models of bewildering complexity, which produce results of implausible precision.'[24] It is certainly true that, since the techniques of meta-analysis first began to emerge in the 1970s, they have been refined into a somewhat arcane art form. Yet the fundamental idea that rigorous numerical methods should be used in summarising the results of clinical trials is surely sound.

Nevertheless, there is a delicious irony about the search for ever greater evidential support in medicine that is behind the rise of meta-analysis. The discounting of anecdotal evidence is certainly in accord with the spirit of science. When the Royal Society, Britain's premier scientific institution, was founded in 1662, it adopted as its motto the Latin phrase *Nullius in verba* – nothing by word alone. Rejecting the deference to authority that had stifled the advance of knowledge for so long, the motto nicely sums up the emphasis on experiment and observation that lies at the heart of the scientific endeavour. Yet in those days it was much simpler for scientists to observe things for themselves. There were only a handful of them, so they could all fit quite comfortably in the same room, and witness important experiments directly. It seemed as if the vagaries and Chinese whispers that beset the reliance on word of mouth had been forever vanquished. The old days, when knowledge was all about scholarship – reporting and commenting on the reports and commentaries of others – had been superseded by an insistence on first-hand observation.

Today we seem to have come full circle. The new regents of medical research can compile their meta-analyses without putting a foot outside their office, let alone actually speaking to a real patient. The papers that sit at the top of the hierarchy of evidence are works of pure scholarship, reports of reports. The 'methods' section contains, not a description of a laboratory procedure, but a string of terms that make up the 'search strategy' used to extract references to medical papers from one or more of the huge electronic databases, such as Medline, that are the present-day equivalent of the vast medieval libraries. And the conclusions of these papers must clearly be taken on trust, as it is impossible for every reader – busy consultants and harried doctors – to check the sources for himself.

Beecher's infamous 1955 paper on the 'powerful placebo' is a case in point. Although lacking the sophisticated statistical apparatus of current meta-analyses, it contains the seeds of the modern idea. It collects a set of clinical trials – no mean feat in those days, when clinical trials themselves were relatively few and far between – and extracts one or two simple figures which everybody remembers. A placebo effect of 35 per cent! This astonishing figure soon became set in stone, transformed into truth by dint of repetition, quoted and requoted by hundreds of doctors who never read Beecher's paper, let alone the studies which he reported. The experimental evidence was trumped by the word of authority, in a parody of the whole enterprise of scientific research. The founders of the Royal Society would have turned in their graves.

Chapter 2

WHAT CAN PLACEBOS REALLY DO?

Dramatic claims have been made for placebos. According to Dr Robert Buckman and Karl Sabbagh, 'they seem to have some effect on almost every symptom known to mankind'.[1] At the other extreme there are those who argue that the placebo effect is largely or even totally illusory. Arthur Shapiro, who spent forty years researching the topic from the mid-1950s until his death in 1995, concluded that there was little evidence for the view that placebos could have a direct and permanent effect on medical disorders.[2] Gunver Kienle and Helmut Kiene have probed the literature on placebos in great depth and found it to be full of misquotation, blind repetition of poorly substantiated claims and the uncritical reporting of anecdotes.[3] The placebo effect, they claim, is no more than a myth.

So much for the claims; what of the evidence? It is true that placebos have been used in thousands of clinical trials, but – as we saw in the last chapter – most of these studies do not include a no-treatment group. As a result, we cannot be sure that the placebo made any difference. The improvement shown by the patients in the placebo group might have occurred anyway as they recovered their health naturally, even if they hadn't received a dummy treatment. To discover what medical conditions the placebo response can really affect, we need to look at the research much more carefully. Only if it can be shown that people with a particular condition do better when treated with a placebo than when not treated at all can we be sure that the placebo response really works for that condition.

THE POWERLESS PLACEBO

In the late 1990s, two medical researchers at the University of Copenhagen attempted to settle the debate about the placebo effect once and for all. Asbjorn Hrobjartsson and Peter Gotzsche combed through the medical literature much more extensively than anyone had done before, picking out all the studies they could find that included both a placebo group and a no-treatment group.[4] They were able to identify a surprisingly large number of such trials – 130 in all. Of these, 114 provided relevant data enabling a proper comparison of the placebo group with the no-treatment group. Using meta-analysis, Hrobjartsson and Gotzsche pooled the results of these studies and concluded that, overall, there was little evidence that placebos had any powerful clinical effects.

This simple conclusion was seized on by the media and reported as proof that the placebo effect was a myth. If they had read the whole study, however, they might not have been so quick to buy Hrobjartsson and Gotzsche's take-home message. The devil, as always, was in the details. For one thing, the studies examined by Hrobjartsson and Gotzsche fell into two distinct groups. Some had reported their results in binary terms (such as positive versus negative result), while others had used a continuous scale (such as the amount of pain relief). For the binary group, there was a small placebo effect, but the result was not significant by the normal standards of statistical research. So far, then, Hrobjartsson and Gotzsche were justified in saying that there was little evidence that placebos had any effect. For the studies using continuous measures, however, there *was* a significant beneficial placebo effect. These studies, then, *do* provide good evidence that placebos can produce clinical benefits.

Furthermore, the range of medical problems covered by the 114 studies analysed by Hrobjartsson and Gotzsche was enormous. In total, forty clinical conditions were examined, from asthma and smoking to menopause, marital discord and schizophrenia. Hrobjartsson and Gotzsche averaged over all these studies and, because there were relatively few in this sample that provided evidence in favour of the placebo effect, the negative view prevailed. But if you did the same thing for virtually any powerful drug, the result would be the same. This is because any kind of therapy that works – be it a drug, a surgical intervention or behavioural therapy – will help people with some conditions and not others. There is no such thing as a universal remedy, a real-life cure-all, a *panacea*.

Certainly, some people have claimed that placebos are just this. Beecher was largely responsible for floating the idea that placebos can affect virtually every medical condition. Although the evidence on which he based this claim was – as we have seen – deeply flawed, the myth of the all-powerful placebo soon became the established medical wisdom. If Hrobjartsson and Gotzsche had contented themselves with exposing this myth, the path would have been opened for a more realistic assessment of the placebo effect, distinguishing between those conditions that are placebo-responsive and those that are not. But Hrobjartsson and Gotzsche went further, asserting that there was no evidence that placebos had any effects at all.

This, at least was the upshot of their brief conclusion. In the small print, however, they were forced to concede that in some cases there were noticeable placebo effects. For some conditions such as anxiety the results were too variable to allow a simple interpretation. For all sorts of pain, however, there was clear positive evidence of a significant placebo effect. Headaches, postoperative pain and sore knees could all be relieved by a sugar pill. There was, then, some reason to suspect that, in pooling the results of studies involving so many different kinds of medical condition, the true profile of the placebo response was obscured.

The mismatch between the complexity of the data analysed by Hrobjartsson and Gotzsche and the stark simplicity of their conclusion is yet another reminder of the need for caution in getting to grips with the research on placebos. What promised to be the final, definitive word on placebos turned out to be a poor study, full of flaws and capped by an inaccurate summary. If we are to get a good idea of what placebos work for – if, indeed, they work for anything – it seems we must go back to square one again, and look at the evidence bit by bit. Only in this way, proceeding carefully, can we begin to build up a picture of what placebos can really do.

NATURAL BORN PAINKILLERS

'To talk about placebos,' writes the American gastroenterologist Howard Spiro, 'is to talk in large part about pain.'[5] Of all the claims made for the placebo response, those that emphasise its power to relieve pain are the most well-established. The pioneers of placebo research focused almost exclusively on the pain-killing properties of placebos. Most of the studies conducted by Beecher, Lasagna and others in the late 1940s and early 1950s were marred, however, by their failure to include no-treatment groups. Typically, they would report that a certain number of patients experienced pain relief after being given a placebo, and conclude that this had been caused by the placebo. This conclusion cannot be trusted, since no attempt was made to measure the spontaneous improvement in patients who did not receive a placebo.

Fortunately, more recent studies of placebo analgesia have included no-treatment control groups in addition to the experimental group and the placebo group. In most of these studies, the no-treatment group has been found to do significantly worse than both the experimental and the placebo groups. We can be confident, then, that the pain reduction experienced by those given the placebo would not simply have happened anyway. Placebo analgesia is real.

In a particularly striking study, patients who had undergone tooth extraction were treated with ultrasound to reduce the postoperative pain.[6] Unknown to both doctors and patients, the experimenters had fiddled with the machine, and half the patients never received the ultrasound. Since ultrasound consists of sound waves of very high frequency – so high, in fact, that they are inaudible to the human ear – there was no way for the doctors or the patients to tell whether or not the machine was emitting the sound waves; the test was truly double-blind. After their jaws were massaged with the ultrasound applicator, the patients were asked to indicate their level of pain on a line where one end was labelled 'no pain' and the other 'unbearable pain'. Compared with the untreated control group, all those treated with the ultrasound machine reported a significant reduction in pain. Surprisingly, it didn't seem to matter whether the machine had been switched on or not. Those who had been massaged with the machine while it was turned off showed the same level of pain reduction as those who had received the proper treatment. In fact, when the ultrasound machine was turned up high, it was actually reported as giving less pain relief than when it was switched off.

We cannot be absolutely sure, even with this model study, that the greater relief experienced by those receiving the fake ultrasound, compared to those receiving no treatment, was due entirely to the placebo effect. Before the switched-off ultrasound machine was applied to the patient's jaw, a coupling cream was rubbed on the skin around it, and this may have reduced the postoperative swelling by itself. Another study examined this possibility by including a control group of patients who were instructed to apply the facial massage, including the cream, to themselves.[7] No reduction in the pain or swelling occurred in this group. The reduction in swelling could not, therefore, have been due to either the massage or the cream. It must have been due to the placebo effect.

Another study to include a no-treatment group compared the placebo response with the powerful painkilling drug bu-prenorphine.[8] Fifty-seven patients with lung cancer who had undergone the notoriously painful operation of thoracotomoy (surgical opening of the chest cavity) and lobectomy (removal of part of the lung) were given injections of buprenorphine at thirty-minute intervals until the pain was adequately reduced. The next day, when their pain had returned to a high level, some of the patients were injected with salt water, while the rest were given no treatment at all. Those who received the saline injection experienced a significant decrease in pain over the following hour, while the pain level of the no-treatment group actually *increased* during the same period. Once again, the body had been encouraged by a pharmacologically inert substance to suppress its own pain.

KINDS OF PAIN

To say that placebos can relieve pain is to make a very general claim. For the species of pain are as abundant as the flora and fauna in a tropical rainforest. Pain can be flickering, quivering, beating or pounding. It can be sharp and cutting or dull and throbbing. It can be caused by material objects such as stinging nettles and bullets, or by tension and worry. There are mild pains, annoying pains, and excruciating pains. And pain can strike anywhere in the body; there are headaches, stomach-aches, swollen ankles, and backaches. It would be impressive indeed if placebos could affect all these different beasts.

Without doing separate tests for each different kind of pain, we cannot be absolutely sure that placebos can relieve them all. However, nobody has yet identified a kind of pain that is completely unresponsive to placebos, which does suggest that they work across the board. The pain of a headache is typically very different to that experienced in the aftermath of a dental operation or chest surgery, yet headaches too are placebo-responsive. In one experiment, two British psychologists recruited over eight hundred female volunteers to take part in a study of headache pills.[9] They gave the volunteers, at random, identical packets of pills, and told them to take two tablets for any headache they had during the following two weeks – and to note down how much relief they obtained. Half the tablets were placebos.

This study did not include a no-treatment group, but it got round this problem in an ingenious way, by making half the packets identical in every way to those of a well-known pain-killer, while the remaining packets were simply labelled 'analgesic tablets'. This applied to both the placebo packets and the packets containing the active tablets, which were of the same well-known brand. There were, therefore, four groups in the study: two placebo groups (one of which was issued with the placebo tablets in a branded packet) and two nonplacebo groups (with the same division into branded and unbranded packets).

By comparing the pain relief from all four groups, the experimenters were able to calculate the effects of branding itself on the treatment of headaches. The result was clear: within each group (placebo and nonplacebo), those taking branded tablets got more relief than those taking unbranded pills – though the branding effect was not as powerful as the effect of the active ingredient. Since branding must clearly act via a psychological route, this study supports the idea that headaches are no exception to the general rule that placebos can affect all sorts of pain.

ALL IN THE MIND?

Placebos are good at reducing pain. But if this were all they were good for, the placebo response could perhaps be dismissed as a mere figment of the patient's imagination. Western medicine distinguishes between symptoms, which are subjective feelings reported by the patient, and signs, which are objective indications of disease detectable by the physician. Pain is, of course, a symptom and not a sign; it cannot be measured by any physical test. The only way, in fact, that we can tell how much pain someone feels is by asking them. All the studies that document placebo analgesia are constrained by this important limitation. They may use various different techniques to gauge the level of pain, from simple yes–no questions to numerical charts on which patients are asked to indicate their current degree of suffering on a scale of zero to ten, but they all have to take the patient's word for it. Is the placebo response, then, just a private affair, dwelling entirely inside the patient's mind?

Some early studies appeared to suggest that this was in fact the case. Two of the most famous, both conducted in the late 1950s, were designed to investigate the effectiveness of an operation known as internal mammary ligation, which was widely practised at the time as a treatment for angina pectoris. Angina is characterised by a vice-like pain in the centre of the chest which tends to be brought on by exercise and goes away with rest. It is generally attributed to the clogging up of the coronary arteries, which reduces the amount of blood these arteries can then supply to the muscle in the heart wall. Internal mammary ligation involved, paradoxically, blocking some of the furred-up arteries completely – the rationale being that the blood would be forced to find alternative routes by sprouting new channels through the heart muscle. These new channels would be free of blockages, and so the circulation in the heart would improve – or so the surgeons hoped. Thousands of operations were carried out without any proof that the new channels did actually sprout, although thousands of patients reported that they felt much better after receiving the operation. Only when pathologists failed to detect any of the supposed new blood vessels in those who had received the operation did some doctors begin to wonder if it had the effect they thought it did.

Two groups of doctors decided to investigate by carrying out controlled trials comparing internal mammary ligation with a placebo operation.[10] This 'sham surgery' involved cutting into the chest and exposing the arteries, but not ligating them. Much to their surprise, the doctors found that patients receiving the dummy operation showed about the same level of improvement as those receiving the real one. The reaction of the medical community was depressingly predictable: instead of being struck by the power of the placebo response, doctors quickly dropped the operation of internal mammary ligation. Nobody paused to wonder how the mere *belief* that one had received a proper operation could be so effective at reducing chest pain.

Of course, without a no-treatment control group, we cannot be sure that the improvement that occurred after these operations was the result of the placebo response, or whether it was simply the natural course of the disease. However, the success rates were high enough to suggest that the placebo response was playing an important role. Around three quarters of all patients reported significantly lower levels of pain, showed a great increase in their exercise tolerance, and decreased their consumption of vasodilating drugs. This is almost certainly a lot more improvement than doctors would expect in the absence of any treatment.

It is important to note, however, that the placebo response – if such it was – did not, in this case, reverse the underlying pathology. No new arteries sprouted in either the experimental group or the placebo group. True, there was an improvement in some 'objective' measures, such as walking distance and drug consumption, but both of these effects could have been due simply to the reduction in pain that followed both the real and the sham operations. A person who feels less pain when exercising can do more before he feels like stopping, and will consume fewer pills; there is nothing mysterious about that. These early studies, then, lend support to the view that placebos can affect symptoms but are powerless to cure disease – they may make you *feel* better, but they don't make you *get* better.

More recent studies of treatments for angina reveal a similar pattern. The main surgical operation for angina today is the coronary-artery bypass graft, in which small sections of vein are removed from the leg and grafted onto the coronary arteries to allow the blood to bypass the blocked areas. This operation does improve survival in the rare cases when the blockage is very serious, but in the majority of less serious cases it has no effect on life expectancy. In fact, when dye is injected into the blood vessels of these patients with less severe cases of angina, it is often found that the new grafts soon become blocked themselves. Surprisingly, though, many of these patients still report a significant reduction in pain.[11] Is the placebo response, then, an entirely subjective phenomenon, as some have claimed?

Beecher and other pioneers of placebo research argued otherwise, but their data was not conclusive. They claimed that patients given placebos showed objective changes, such as constricted pupils, but they could not prove that these changes were directly attributable to the placebo response because their studies did not include no-treatment control groups. The sceptic could always argue that such objective changes might have occurred anyway. One early study went some way to meeting this objection by using a patient as his own control.[12] A man with a hole in his stomach was tested for the level of gastric acid after being treated with a placebo, and the results were compared with his reactions at other times when no treatment was administered. The gastric acid level fell twice as often when a placebo was used as when no agent was administered. The sceptic could still object, however, since the sample size was so small: only one patient, and only twenty-six observations.

Fortunately, more recent studies have produced much stronger evidence. The studies that looked at the effect of ultrasound on postoperative dental pain, for example, found that objective measures were also affected by the placebo response.[13] Not only did those who received the fake ultrasound (while the machine was switched off) experience a reduction in pain, but in one of the studies trismus was also significantly reduced compared to the no-treatment control group. Trismus is an involuntary contraction of the jaw muscles which keeps the jaw tightly closed – and can be measured objectively. Furthermore, in both of the studies there was also a significant decrease in swelling in those receiving the fake ultrasound. Inflammation is even less of a 'mental' process than trismus. The placebo response is clearly not just a subjective affair.

ULCERS

The fact that trismus and inflammation can be affected by dummy treatments shows that the placebo response is not limited to subjective symptoms. Nevertheless, if these were the *only* objective signs that placebos could affect, it would be a hollow victory for the placebo response, falling far short of dramatic claims such as that cited at the beginning of this chapter. Inflammation and involuntary muscular spasms may well be objective signs of pathology, but they are not particularly dangerous problems. Is there any evidence that placebos can affect more serious conditions?

There is. Daniel Moerman, a medical anthropologist at the University of Michigan, has provided persuasive evidence that placebos can cure ulcers. Moerman began by gathering the results of seventy-one controlled trials of drugs for treating stomach ulcers. As usual, these studies did not include no-treatment groups, and so no individual trial provided direct evidence of a placebo response. By examining the studies together, however, Moerman was able to detect a pattern that did suggest that the placebos were having a powerful effect. Ingeniously, he compared those studies in which patients took *two* placebos a day to those in which patients took *four* placebos a day. In the first group, 33 per cent were healed, while in the second, 38 per cent were healed.[14] This might not seem like a big difference, but it is statistically significant, and it has been replicated in another, more rigorous meta-analysis.[15]

Comparing two groups of patients taking different amounts of placebos is almost as good, scientifically speaking, as comparing a placebo group with a no-treatment group. The fact that those taking more placebos showed more improvement strongly suggests that the placebos were playing an active role in assisting recovery. Furthermore, the improvement was not just subjective. All the studies examined by Moerman checked whether the ulcers had really healed by using an endoscope to peer inside the patients' stomachs.

PLACEBOS AND MENTAL DISORDER

What about mental disorders? Can placebos cure diseases of the mind as well as diseases of the body? Unfortunately, the available evidence is once again quite weak. Despite the oft-repeated claims in the medical literature about 'well-documented' placebo effects in anxiety and depression, there are no properly controlled studies showing that people with these conditions do better when given a placebo than when deprived of one. In the absence of such studies, we can still look for relevant evidence by sifting through other data and comparing one set of trials with another, but we should bear in mind that the conclusions we draw on this basis must always be treated with a degree of caution. Until someone comes along and does a proper study involving a no-treatment group, it would be wrong to say that the placebo response has been clearly demonstrated for anxiety and depression.

Although there are a few controlled trials comparing placebos to no treatment with patients suffering from various anxiety disorders, these suffer from methodological flaws and do not provide very strong evidence. There are other kinds of evidence, however, which – while by no means conclusive – do provide some basis for suspecting that placebos can reduce anxiety. One study, for example, looked at the effect of tablet colour in the treatment of anxiety states.[16] In 1970, a group of researchers based at the University of Newcastle upon Tyne signed up forty-eight patients who had been diagnosed as suffering from anxiety states, and divided them into three groups. All of the patients received a course of oxazepam, which is a cousin of diazepam (Valium), but the pills given to each group were dyed with a different colour – red, yellow and green. The colours were switched around after a week, and then switched once more for the third week, so that each group tried each colour. Anxiety levels were monitored both subjectively (by self-assessment forms) and objectively (by the doctors – who were unaware of which colour pill the patient was taking at any particular time).

When the results came in, some interesting trends were apparent in the data. The colour of the tablets seemed to have a subtle influence on the effect of the medication. In particular, green tablets tended to be most effective in reducing anxiety, and yellow the least effective. Anxiety manifests itself in a number of ways, from psychological symptoms such as worry and irritability to bodily signs such as palpitations, and for all of these phenomena green tablets were superior to the red or yellow ones. The differences were small, though, and did not reach statistical significance, except in one case – phobic symptoms. Phobia is one of the most common manifestations of anxiety, and green tablets were twice as effective as red or yellow ones in reducing phobic symptoms – even though the tablets contained exactly the same drug.

When the effect of a drug varies systematically according to colour of the tablet in which it is administered, it is a fair bet that the condition being treated is placebo-responsive. The only way that something as insubstantial as colour can affect a medical condition is by way of the patient's mind. The 1970 study on tablet colour does therefore suggest that some anxiety disorders at least may be placebo-responsive. Interestingly, the same study also pointed to a possible placebo effect in depression. This is not particularly surprising in itself, since anxiety and depressive symptoms often occur together, but the curious thing was that the best colour for treating each type of symptom was different. While anxiety levels were reduced most by green tablets, depressive symptoms responded best to yellow tablets. Next best was green, while red was worst for both anxiety and depression. The researchers who conducted the study were at a loss to explain this result. Was it due to chance? Or did it point to certain differences in the patients' beliefs about the effects of tablet colour? Intrigued, they called for further research on the topic. None came.

WHAT ABOUT DEPRESSION?

Although the 1970 study on tablet colour suggested that depression, too, was placebo-responsive, hard data is thin on the ground. Hundreds of clinical trials have compared the effects of antidepressant medication with those of placebos, but none has included a no-placebo group. In the absence of such studies, we cannot be sure whether or not depression is placebo-responsive. In 1998, however, two American psychologists, Irving Kirsch and Guy Sapirstein, came up with an ingenious way round this problem. None of the drug trials they looked at included a no-treatment control group, but a whole batch of studies of *psychotherapeutic* treatments did. Many of these studies, for example, compared the recovery rates of depressed patients receiving psychotherapy with the recovery rates of other depressed patients who remained on waiting lists. Kirsch and Sapirstein used the waiting-list recovery rate as a rough measure of the spontaneous remission rate, and compared it with the recovery rate shown by those taking placebos in the drug trials. In this way, they were able to estimate the relative effects of placebos and antidepressant drugs. Their conclusions were startling. Those taking drugs showed, on average, about 33 per cent more improvement than those treated with a placebo. But those taking a placebo showed around 200 per cent more improvement than those who received no treatment at all. If we assume that the placebo component of the real drug is the same as that of the pure placebo, then we must conclude that around 25 per cent of the improvement shown by those taking antidepressants is due to spontaneous remission, 50 per cent to the placebo effect, and only a measly 25 per cent to the antidepressant medication itself.[17]

Donald Klein, a psychiatrist at Columbia University in New York, has cast doubt on this dramatic conclusion.[18] Klein argues that many of the studies on which Kirsch and Sapirstein based their claims were flawed for various reasons. More importantly, Klein also raises questions about the scales used to measure recovery. A typical five-point scale might go something like this:

1 = normal functioning
2 = mild functional impairment
3 = definitely impaired
4 = cannot work
5 = impaired self-care

Now, suppose that all the patients in a trial start out at a mean of 4.5 on this scale – they cannot work, and some of them cannot even take care of themselves properly. If the average patient on medication improves by three points, and the average patient on placebo improves by 2.25 points, Kirsch and Sapirstein would argue that for the typical patient, 75 per cent of the drug effect is attributable to the placebo effect, which makes the superiority of the drug seem relatively trivial. If, however, we look at where the patients end up on the scale, the superiority of the drug begins to look more important, for the average patient on medication is now between normal functioning and mild impairment, while the average patient on placebo is now between mild and definite impairment. This difference is clinically important, and yet it is hidden by the way that Kirsch and Sapirstein report the data.

On the other hand, it may be that the placebo effect in depression is even greater than Kirsch and Sapirstein claim. As they themselves point out, the placebo component of a real drug may be higher than the placebo effect of a pure placebo. Placebo effects depend in large part on the belief that you are being given an effective treatment, and there is evidence that many participants in clinical trials guess correctly whether they are receiving the real drug or the placebo. The real drug tends to have noticeable side-effects that the placebo lacks. In one study comparing two antidepressants (imipramine and phenelzine) with a placebo, 78 per cent of patients and 87 per cent of psychiatrists correctly guessed who was receiving an active drug and who was receiving the placebo.[19] In fact, in twenty-three out of twenty-six studies where researchers bothered to check, both patients and physicians did better than chance at guessing who was receiving the placebo and who was not.[20]

If patients guess they are taking a placebo, this may reduce the power of the placebo to unleash their internal healing resources. On the other hand, if they guess they are taking the experimental drug, this might enhance the placebo effect. Arguing along these lines, Kirsch and Sapirstein suggested that some of the apparent difference between real drugs and pure placebos may be due to an 'enhanced placebo effect'. If this is true, the ratio of the specific effect of the real drug to its placebo component becomes even smaller still.

To disentangle the true specific effect of a treatment not only from spontaneous remission and the effect of a pure placebo such as a sugar pill, but also from the enhanced placebo effect of the real drug, Kirsch and Sapirstein suggest that clinical trials should involve not two arms, as most do at present, nor even three, but *four*. In addition to the experimental group, the no-treatment group and the pure placebo group, a fourth arm would treat patients with a so-called 'active placebo'. This is a placebo that lacks the key ingredient of the experimental treatment but contains some other active substance designed to produce similar side-effects. Some trials of antidepressants, for example, have used atropine as an active placebo because it produces one of the most noticeable side-effects that many anti-depressants do – a dry mouth – but does not have any specific activity against depression itself. Needless to say, such four-arm trials are even less common than three-arm trials. In fact, they are virtually non-existent at present. They would, however, be invaluable in advancing our understanding of the placebo phenomenon.

A few clinical trials of antidepressant drugs have used active placebos instead of pure placebos. That is, they have compared two groups of patients – one that receives the experimental drug, and one that is given an active placebo such as atropine.

These trials reduce the chances that the double-blind will be broken – in other words, they make it harder for patients or their doctors to guess who is receiving the experimental drug and who is receiving the placebo. Interestingly, these trials tend to show much lower drug effects than those in which anti-depressants are compared to pure placebos.[21] This, in itself, provides some evidence for a placebo effect in depression. The argument is a subtle one, but worth exploring.

If depression was not placebo-responsive, then the whole effect of antidepressant drugs would be due to the pharmacological properties of the drugs themselves. It would make no difference whether you believed you were taking the drug or not. The difference in recovery rates between patients taking the drug and patients taking placebos would therefore be the same whether or not patients were able to guess correctly which group they were in. This is not, however, what we find. When patients are able to guess which group they are in, the difference between the experimental group and the placebo group increases. This suggests that belief is indeed playing some role in the efficacy of antidepressant medication. The placebo effect, in other words, does seem to work for depression.

PLACEBOS AND SCHIZOPHRENIA

If placebos worked for every kind of mental disorder, their power would not be limited to anxiety and depression, but would extend even to the most severe psychoses, including schizophrenia. Is there any evidence that placebos can affect such extreme mental conditions?

In the 1950s, many psychiatrists were unwilling to accept the idea that placebos could alleviate depression, let alone schizophrenia. One German psychiatrist, however, decided to test the idea. Heinz Lehmann picked three of the most mute and deteriorated schizophrenics on one of the back wards at Verdun hospital. He told the patients and their nurses that they were going to try out a new experimental hormone, which was, in fact, just a placebo. The injection site was painted with a disinfectant that left a prominent red stain, and the patients were injected twice a week for two weeks. By the third week, two of the three had broken their silence, and were talking quite sensibly.[22]

This study is, as far as I can tell, the only evidence that schizophrenia might be placebo-responsive, and it is not particularly strong evidence at that. For a start, there was no control group, the sample size was tiny – only three patients – and we do not know how long the improvement lasted. We cannot even be sure that the three patients were all really suffering from schizophrenia. Back in the 1950s, diagnostic standards were extremely variable, and the diagnosis of schizophrenia in particular was often used as a catch-all category to deal with any kind of patient whose prognosis was not good. Many people with learning disabilities, personality disorders or even simply unconventional behaviour were tagged as schizophrenics and confined to locked wards throughout Europe and America, where they eventually became so institutionalised that their behaviour mimicked the very diagnosis they had been given. They became mute and withdrawn, just as those suffering from the catatonic form of schizophrenia were supposed to. A vicious circle would establish itself, in which the condition of the patients and the pessimistic views of the nursing staff regarding their recovery became mutually reinforcing. It is not hard to see how, given a change in the views of the nursing staff, this circle could be broken. Perhaps this is what occurred with Lehmann's patients. If so, it is not really a case of placebos curing schizophrenia.

In the absence of more conclusive evidence, then, it would be premature to pronounce any verdict on whether or not placebos can affect severe psychotic illnesses such as schizophrenia. For the time being, all we can say is that less serious mental conditions such as anxiety disorders and most types of depression do appear to be placebo-responsive. When it comes to schizophrenia, the jury is still out.

THE LIMITS OF THE PLACEBO RESPONSE

Tracing the limits of the placebo response is not easy. So far, we have seen that there is good evidence that it works for pain and some of the minor signs of injury, such as inflammation and trismus. There is also some evidence that placebos can alleviate depression and anxiety and cure ulcers. On the other hand, there is no real evidence that the placebo response can do anything to reverse cancer or cure schizophrenia. It would be interesting to know if there is any underlying logic to this. What is it that determines whether or not a medical condition responds to a placebo?

To answer this question, we must delve deeper into the underlying mechanisms of the placebo response. The placebo response is simply a rapid readjustment of the body's own natural healing mechanisms to a surge of hope, and there are limits to what these mechanisms can do, even if fuelled with industrial-strength optimism. The placebo response is not magic; it works by natural mechanisms, and all such mechanisms have their limits. These mechanisms are the subject of the following chapter.

Chapter 3

THE ACUTE PHASE RESPONSE

It is all very well to know which conditions placebos can affect and which they can't, but a good scientific theory requires more than just a list. Chemistry, for example, only became a true science when the great Russian chemist Dmitri Mendeleyev took the list of known elements and perceived a hidden pattern in the data. The periodic table, which Mendeleyev first formulated in 1869, made this pattern visible to all, and allowed scientists to uncover the fundamental order that underlay the mass of empirical results that they had accumulated in the previous centuries. To put the placebo response on an equally scientific footing, we must look beneath the signs and symptoms described in the previous chapter and ask whether there is some mechanism, or set of mechanisms, which explains why placebos can do the things they can, and why they can't do the things they can't.

At first sight, the list of conditions that placebos can alleviate may appear an odd bunch, lacking any common thread, as random as the elements must have appeared to those before Mendeleyev. Recent discoveries in immunology, however, have uncovered strong links between these conditions. It turns out that pain, swelling, stomach ulcers, depression and anxiety do, in fact, have something in common: they all involve the activation of a complex biological phenomenon known as the acute phase response. Perhaps this is the key to understanding the placebo effect.

44

THE ACUTE PHASE RESPONSE

Dealing with injury and infection is vital to survival. It is hardly surprising, then, that all animals possess mechanisms designed specifically to deal with wound healing and microbial defence. In mammals such as ourselves, these mechanisms are remarkably complex and, when they function correctly, produce an exquisitely choreographed suite of reactions which biologists are only now beginning to fully appreciate. The first stage in this process is known as the acute phase response, or, less technically, as inflammation.

For hundreds of years, Western medicine recognised the four signs of inflammation as *tumor, rubor, calor* and *dolor* – swelling, redness, heat and pain. In the last decades of the twentieth century, biologists discovered a few more. Besides these physical changes, there are also important psychological ones, including lethargy, apathy, loss of appetite and increased sensitivity to pain – a suite of symptoms that are collectively known as 'sickness behaviour'.[1] Taken together, the four classic signs of inflammation and the psychological symptoms of sickness behaviour constitute the complex set of processes referred to as the acute phase response.[2]

For a long time, doctors tended to regard the signs of inflammation and sickness behaviour as part of the disease process itself. The lethargy that commonly ensues after infection, for example, was thought to result from debilitation, as if the body had simply run out of energy. It is now known, however, that the various components of the acute phase response are not themselves pathological. On the contrary; they are actively produced by the body itself as part of the healing process. They may feel unpleasant, but they are actually good for you. In fact, feeling unpleasant is a vital part of their function.

PAIN

The value of feeling bad is nowhere better illustrated than in the case of pain. Pain, as everyone knows, is a great protector. The classic textbook illustration shows someone withdrawing their hand very rapidly from a hot stove they have just touched by accident. This acute pain is obviously beneficial, causing you to move away quickly from damaging objects. Even more important, however, is the second phase of pain that tends to follow the acute pain. Acute pain is sharp and stabbing, and ends when you are no longer in contact with the source of damage; the second type of pain is deep and spreading, and can last for minutes, hours, days, or even months. This kind of pain is not caused by pressure or heat from the outside world, but by chemicals released by the body itself. And, unlike acute pain, which produces rapid movement, the second type of pain causes you to keep the wounded area as still as possible, and encourages you to take extra care to shield the area from fresh injury while the process of repair is completed.

The capacity for pain, then, confers an advantage on those who have it. Exactly *how* advantageous this capacity is may be inferred from the sorry fate of those rare individuals who happen to be born without it. Almost everyone with this condition, which is known as congenital analgesia, is dead by the age of thirty. Without the capacity for acute pain, they do not withdraw from damaging objects unless their other senses inform them of the injury. One girl with the disorder, for example, knelt on a hot radiator while she gazed out of a window, blissfully unaware of the burning flesh. Her knees were scarred for the rest of her life, which was not very long, since she died at the age of twenty-two.[3]

It is not the lack of *acute* pain that kills people with congenital analgesia, however, but the lack of the second kind of pain. The lack of the deeper, longer-lasting second phase of pain is far more deadly than the lack of acute pain, since no effort is made to guard wounded areas. The result is that injuries never heal properly, and the accumulating mass of dead and damaged tissue becomes a target for bacteria, which eat their way into the bone marrow. Having bacteria inside your bones is a serious condition called osteomyelitis; this was what eventually killed the girl who knelt on the radiator.

Next time you are gripped by an intense pain, then, you might pause to consider how lucky you are. Evolution has endowed you with a vital defence mechanism, and without it your life expectancy would be considerably shorter. In a world where minor injuries such as scratches, burns, and bruises are common fare, it really is good to be able to feel bad.

SWELLING

The same logic applies to all the other aspects of the acute phase response. Swelling, for example, is also a defensive process, caused by the leakage of plasma and the migration of immune cells into the area of damaged tissue. All bodily damage, whether caused by injury or infection, consists of broken cells, and when the walls of a cell rupture, an array of molecules, which would not otherwise be released, spill out into the surrounding tissue. Some of these molecules trigger the sensory nerves to produce the ongoing, second type of pain just described. The sensory nerves also react by causing the blood vessels to widen, increasing local blood flow, and making the walls of the blood vessels more permeable. With greater blood flow, more white blood cells – the infantry of the immune system – can be carried to the site of the injury. The greater permeability of the blood-vessel walls enables the white blood cells to flow out of the arteries and veins into the surrounding tissue to defend against possible bacterial invaders. If no bacteria have found their way into the wound, particular white blood cells known as macrophages clear up the debris of the shattered cells by engulfing and digesting it. If bacteria have gained a foothold and started to multiply, the white cells form a barrier to create a pus-filled abscess in which the blood fluid – the serum – plays a key role in healing.

Besides clearing up debris and attacking bacteria themselves, the macrophages also release a number of chemical messengers. These signalling molecules, or cytokines, play a vital role in co-ordinating the acute phase response by facilitating both short-distance communication among the immune cells themselves, and long-distance communication between the immune cells at the injured site and the brain.

Many different cytokines are involved in the acute phase response, but one seems to play a starring role. Known as inter-leukin-1ß (IL-1ß), it is one of the first cytokines to be released by the macrophages on detecting signs of injury or infection. The IL-1ß diffuses into the tissue surrounding the damaged cells, where it triggers a second wave of cytokines which cause other types of immune cell such as neutrophils and monocytes to migrate to the injured site.[4] The IL-1ß released by the macrophages also enters the bloodstream, where it is carried to the brain, but is prevented from entering the brain directly by a layer of cells known as the blood-brain barrier. It therefore adopts a more cunning route into the central nervous system.[5] First, the IL-1ß molecules attach themselves to specially-designed receptors on the surface of the cells in the blood-brain barrier. When these receptors are activated, a chain reaction is initiated that eventually leads to the manufacture of a molecule known as prostaglandin E2, which – unlike IL-1ß – is capable of passing through the blood-brain barrier. When it enters the brain, prostaglandin E2 activates receptors on both neurons and microglia (immune cells in the brain), which can then initiate the other components of the acute phase response: fever, lethargy, apathy, loss of appetite, anxiety, and increased sensitivity to pain in other areas of the body. But the story does not end there. Once inside the brain, prostaglandin E2 encourages the microglia to manufacture IL-1ß. The net result is that, although IL-1ß cannot cross the blood-brain barrier directly, a build-up of IL-1ß in the bloodstream leads to a build-up of IL-1ß in the brain and the cerebrospinal fluid. To complete the cycle, the IL-1ß leads to further synthesis of prostaglandin E2 in the brain, which in turn augments the various components of sickness behaviour.

FEVER

Increasing levels of prostaglandin E2 in the brain induce an area called the hypothalamus to turn up the body's thermostat a notch. Suddenly, the same external temperature feels colder, and various means are employed to restore the subjective impression of warmth. These include involuntary processes such as shivering, which generates heat by movement, and voluntary behaviour such as putting on more clothes, finding a warm radiator to sit next to, and so on.

Like pain and swelling, fever plays a vital part in defending the body against infection. Many bacteria that infect humans reproduce most effectively at normal human body temperature, so by raising body temperature, the rate at which the bacteria can divide is slowed down.[6] Fever has the opposite effect on most immune cells, causing them to divide more quickly. So fever both slows down the spread of the infection, and accelerates the counter-attack by the immune system.

Blocking fever with drugs interferes with this part of the healing process, and can lead to dangerous consequences. Experiments have shown that when infected animals are treated with antipyretics (drugs that reduce fever), they are more likely to die from the infection.[7] Sometimes, the fever can get out of control, in which case antipyretics can save lives, but when the fever is not too high, it is probably better not to block it artificially. As with the other components of the acute phase response, fever may feel unpleasant, but it plays a vital role in the healing process.

LETHARGY, APATHY AND LOSS OF APPETITE

Fever is not cheap. The body has to work incredibly hard to raise its temperature. In mammals, an increase of just one degree celsius in core body temperature requires around 10–13 per cent more energy than normal.[8] To balance the energy budget, savings must therefore be made elsewhere, and the brain accordingly generates feelings of lethargy and apathy which reduce the energy expended in behaviour. Sick people generally do not feel like doing very much, but this is not because they have simply 'run out of energy'. They are merely saving their energy to use in other ways.

In view of the need for more energy to assist the healing process, the loss of appetite that occurs in response to infection might seem paradoxical. It becomes easier to understand when you remember that we did not evolve in a world of supermarkets and convenience stores. For our ancestors on the African plains, as for so many animals, finding food could be an arduous task, and it may well have been better to avoid the energetic cost of foraging by suppressing hunger rather than using up one's valuable calories by looking for more food. Besides, hunting and foraging also expose one to the risk of more infection and injury, which could be doubly dangerous to an organism that is already damaged.

The loss of appetite in the acute phase response may also be accompanied by feelings of nausea, which may even lead to the loss of precious food by vomiting. This seems even more paradoxical than loss of appetite, in view of the need to conserve energy when one is sick. However, even here there are possible advantages, which include reinforcing the loss of appetite and expelling pathogens and toxins from the stomach. Food represents a problem for the immune system since it is foreign, and yet necessary for survival. The body must constantly replenish itself by converting non-self into self. Certain substances, though, will not do. Sugar and fat are vital sources of energy, but arsenic is not. Distinguishing between foods and toxins is just as vital as distinguishing between good and bad bacteria. The two kinds of threat are dealt with by different means – attacking one and regurgitating the other – but the overall aim is the same.

Like so many other aspects of immune activity, nausea and

vomiting are closely governed by the brain. The plasma cells that line our intestines, ready to churn out antibodies at a moment's notice, respond both to toxins and to psychological input. Stress and anxiety can make you feel sick just as easily as, and much more quickly than, a sandwich past its sell-by date. And, once again, the same signalling molecules seem to be involved: IL-1ß is also known to generate feelings of nausea.

To compensate for the decreased supply of new calories caused by loss of appetite (and possibly the loss of calories by vomiting), the body starts to unleash old calories that have been stored up for just such times of emergency. These calories are stored in fat deposits around the body, but before the fat can be used as a source of energy it must be broken down into glucose. So another crucial component of the acute phase response is the secretion of glucocorticoids, which trigger the process of converting fat to glucose. The key glucocorticoid in humans is cortisol, which is released by the adrenal glands in response to a cascade of chemical signals initiated in the brain by IL-1ß. First, the IL-1ß stimulates the hypothalamus to secrete a chemical called corticotrophin releasing hormone (CRH). The CRH travels to the pituitary gland, just below the brain, where it triggers the release of another chemical called adrenocortico-tropic hormone (ACTH). Finally, the ACTH reaches the adrenal glands, which secrete the cortisol. Because of their close interconnections, the three anatomical structures involved in this chemical cascade are known collectively as the hypothal-amo-pituitary-adrenal axis, or HPA for short.

PLACEBO-RESPONSIVE CONDITIONS AND THE ACUTE PHASE RESPONSE

The details of the acute phase response are much more complex than the brief outline here may suggest. There are, for example, many more cytokines involved than just IL-1ß, and many of these affect other organs in the body besides the brain and the endocrine system. The liver plays a vital role in the acute phase response, supplying molecules known as acute phase proteins, and helping to dispose of harmful agents detected by the immune cells. When one gets down to the level of gene transcription, the details become even more subtle. However, the brief sketch given above will do for now.

If you compare the range of phenomena involved in the acute phase response to the range of placebo-responsive conditions in the last chapter, the similarity may not be obvious at first. Pain, of course, is present in both lists, as is swelling; but what about stomach ulcers, depression and anxiety? These three conditions all respond to placebos, but what have they got to do with the acute phase response? If the claim that placebo-responsive conditions all involve the activation of the acute phase response is to stand up, some further explanation is called for.

Even in the case of pain, it may not be clear that all the sorts of pain that placebos can affect are properly regarded as part of the acute phase response. On the face of it, it appears that many non-inflammatory painful conditions respond to placebos. Many experiments, for example, have induced pain by means of techniques such as electrical and thermal stimulation that do not result in the other components of the acute phase response, yet respond to placebos. There are also other forms of natural pain such as migraine, tension-type headache and many others, that can be alleviated by placebos, yet do not seem to have an inflammatory component. However, while these sorts of pain may not produce visible swelling, inflammation may still be involved. The inflammatory process was first identified by doctors thousands of years ago by means of obvious visible signs such as redness and swelling, but the underlying causes of these signs have only been discovered in the past few decades. The cytokines that control the whole process interact in complex ways that may result in the suppression of the traditional signs of inflammation while generating other symptoms that have only recently been recognised as playing an equally important part in the acute phase response – the symptoms of sickness behaviour, for example. So long as these cytokines are activated in all the forms of pain that are placebo-responsive, the claim that placebo-responsive conditions involve the activation of the acute phase response still holds.

Stomach ulcers, too, involve inflammation. An ulcer is a breach in the mucosal lining of the stomach which may be caused by a variety of factors. The discovery, in the 1980s, of a strange corkscrew-shaped bacterium in the stomachs of those with ulcers swept away previous theories about the role of stress and diet, but some researchers now argue that this was an overreaction, and that psychological factors are also involved. Stress may therefore still play a role in explaining why only some people infected with *Helicobacter pylori* go on to develop ulcers. Despite dozens of studies, very little is known about the manner in which *H. pylori* incites or enhances inflammation. IL-1ß is thought to play a key part, along with other cytokines such as IL-6, and this suggests that the acute phase response is somehow activated.

Depression may seem, at first sight, to have little in common with inflammation, but once again, appearances can be misleading. Local inflammation, as we have seen, can trigger a cascade of chemical signals that result in the symptoms of sickness behaviour. These feelings – which include lethargy, apathy, loss of appetite, decreased sexual activity and general malaise – also happen to be the main symptoms of depression. This curious coincidence has not gone unnoticed by doctors, and has even led some to argue that depression may turn out to be an inflammatory disorder.[9] The Belgian immunologist Michael Maes has shown that the same chemical messenger that plays a leading role in exporting local inflammation to the brain and triggering sickness behaviour after infection – IL-1ß – is also produced in greater amounts by macrophages in the blood of severely depressed people.[10] Maes and his team have also found that depressed patients have increased levels of other markers associated with the acute phase response, including various members of the interleukin family (IL-2 receptor and IL-6) and plasma proteins such as haptoglobin. All of this has led Maes to argue that depression is associated with a chronic activation of the acute phase response.

The idea that depression involves an overactive immune response is by no means universally accepted. At present, all the hard data supporting the idea stems from the work of a single research group – that of Michael Maes – and has not yet been replicated by other teams. Until independent studies are done, many immunologists will probably remain sceptical. After all, most previous studies have pointed in the opposite direction, suggesting that depression results in a blunted immune response rather than an overactive one. Many studies, for example, have reported that depressed patients show a reduction in the activity of certain types of white blood cell known as natural killer cells. Nevertheless, there are many confounding factors that may explain the apparently contradictory results obtained so far. To take just one example, depressed people tend to smoke more than those who are not depressed, and it may be that it is the increased level of nicotine consumption that produces some of the altered immune responses associated with depression. Such confounding variables could tip the balance in favour of Maes's theory, or tell against it. The jury is still out, but one thing is clear: the theory that depression involves activation of the acute phase response deserves to be more fully investigated.

Anxiety disorders, too, are bound up with the immune system in similar ways. In phobias and panic attacks the body's natural stress response is pushed into overdrive, and elevated levels of the stress hormone, cortisol, are found in people with these disorders. Increased levels of cortisol are also found in people with depression, which is not surprising given the large overlap between the symptoms of depression and anxiety. Many people with depression experience intermittent bouts of anxiety, and many people with anxiety disorders report long episodes of low mood. In technical terms, there is a high degree of co-morbidity between depression and anxiety. Some researchers have speculated that the depressive states in which anxiety symptoms are also present may constitute a disorder in their own right, distinct from other kinds of depression. If so, this is another possible explanation for the apparently contradictory results that have emerged from studies of immune parameters in depressed patients. Because these studies tend to pool all types of depression together, they may be failing to pick up important differences between one kind of depressive disorder and another.

THE PARADOXES OF CORTISOL

There is something strange about the co-morbidity of depression and anxiety. Michael Maes and his group have found evidence that levels of IL-1ß are increased in depressed patients. The key chemical marker in anxiety, on the other hand, is cortisol. Cortisol is widely supposed to be anti-inflammatory, and most anti-inflammatory drugs contain similar substances. Cortisol is also known to inhibit the expression of the pro-inflammatory cytokine, IL-1ß. So how can high levels of IL-1ß co-exist in depression alongside high levels of cortisol?

One possibility is that the continual output of cortisol in depression can lead the immune system to become desensitised to this hormone. The result is that high levels of cortisol can then co-exist in the body with high levels of IL-1ß, which would not normally be possible. However, it may be that cortisol does not, in fact, inhibit IL-1ß even in the normal person.

Some immunologists claim that, in the normal person, cortisol acts as a negative feedback mechanism, regulating the inflammatory response by keeping levels of IL-1ß under control.[11] It is known that, besides its role in provoking inflammation, IL-1ß also triggers the HPA axis to produce cortisol. This may appear paradoxical, but there are in fact dozens of feedback loops, some positive and some negative, that help the immune system to keep itself in balance. In such feedback loops, the timing of various counter-regulatory signals is essential, and some have suggested that timing is the key to the cortisol circuit. The inflammatory effects of IL-1ß are apparent within minutes, allowing the body to respond very quickly to injury and infection. But IL-1ß takes much longer to get the HPA axis going, so by the time the cortisol arrives on the scene, the inflammatory response is already well in place. The cortisol arrives just in time, it has been suggested, to prevent the inflammatory response from reaching extreme levels. The circuit therefore functions as a negative-feedback loop.

This theory is certainly plausible, but there are also problems with it. Specifically, the amounts of cortisol released by the HPA axis in response to stimulation by IL-1ß are much smaller than those used in anti-inflammatory drugs, and at these levels cortisol may actually enhance inflammation.[12] There are, in fact, various different kinds of inflammation, and cortisol-type drugs may dampen down one kind but stimulate the kind associated with the acute phase response. So, rather than functioning to switch off the acute phase response, low levels of cortisol may actually provide positive feedback that keeps it going. The details are clearly very complex, and it would be premature to pronounce any definitive conclusions. Nevertheless, the evidence is mounting that the same family of closely related mechanisms underlie pain, swelling, ulcers, depression and anxiety. These mechanisms are the very same as those involved in the acute phase response. This suggests that the reason placebos can alleviate some conditions but not others is to be found in the workings of the immune system.

ENDORPHINS

If all the conditions that respond to placebos involve the activation of the acute phase response, then placebos may work by suppressing that response. To find out whether this is in fact what placebos do, we would have to compare the mechanisms activated by placebos with those that suppress the acute phase response. Unfortunately, little is known about either of these things. Nevertheless, there is some evidence that suggests we may be on the right track.

The mechanisms by which placebos achieve their various

effects are still largely obscure, but some progress at least has been made in understanding how they alleviate pain. The story begins in 1978, when an ingenious study conducted by Jon Levine, N.C. Gordon and Howard Fields was published in the *Lancet*.[13] The first part of the study showed a typical placebo response: Levine and his colleagues administered placebo medication to patients with postoperative pain and, sure enough, the usual decrease in pain was observed. At that point, however, the researchers injected the patients with naloxone, after which the pain returned to its previous intensity. Naloxone is an antidote to morphine, and can be used to treat morphine poisoning. But the patients in Levine's study had not been given morphine; they had simply been treated with an inert substance. So what was going on?

Naloxone works by blocking the same receptor sites in the brain which morphine molecules attach themselves to. A few years before Levine's study, scientists had shown that these receptors were also targets for certain naturally-occurring substances in the brain whose chemical structure was similar to that of morphine. They called these natural painkillers 'endorphins' – short for endogenous morphine. Levine argued that naloxone was blocking the placebo response in the same way that it blocked the effects of morphine – by blocking the morphine receptors in the brain – and that endorphins might therefore be the underlying mechanism by which placebos reduced pain.

Many questions remained. For a start, even if placebos did reduce pain by triggering the release of endorphins, it was still unclear how and why that should happen in the first place. By what mechanisms could the injection of an inert substance such as salt water send a message to the pituitary gland to release its natural painkillers? And why was the pituitary not releasing them beforehand, when the patient was in such obvious pain? Despite its failure to address these problems, the Levine paper had a tremendous impact on placebo research. According to the late Patrick Wall, one of the world's leading experts in the understanding of pain, the study 'converted a previously mysterious,

magical phenomenon into one associated with objective pharmacology and therefore made the placebo respectable'.[14]

Attempts to replicate Levine's experiment by other scientists
have produced mixed results. Some studies have confirmed
Levine's findings, while others have found that naloxone has
little or no effect on placebo-induced analgesia. On the whole,
however, evidence is growing that the power of placebos to
reduce pain is due to their ability to unleash the body's own
natural painkillers. But what about the capacity of placebos to
reduce swelling, cure ulcers, and alleviate depression and anxiety? Do they achieve these effects too by triggering the release
of endorphins, or is some other mechanism involved?

A hint that endorphins might also play a part in reducing
swelling was provided by one of the studies on fake ultrasound
that we looked at in the last chapter. We saw there that a team
of dentists found that when they administered a switched-off
ultrasound machine to patients who had just had teeth removed,
both pain and swelling were significantly reduced. In one of
these studies the dentists went on to give the patients a dose
of naloxone.[15] Just as expected, the pain returned – but so also
did the swelling. Naloxone, it seems, does not only abolish
the painkilling effect of placebos; it also reverses their anti-
inflammatory action. This suggests that the power of placebos
to reduce swelling is based on the same mechanism as that
which underlies their power to reduce pain – the release of
endorphins.

Endorphins and other chemical messengers allow the brain
to exert some degree of downward control over pain and the
inflammatory response. It is likely, then, that these are the
physical mechanisms that underlie the analgesic and anti-
inflammatory capacities of placebos. It is still too early to say
whether the same mechanisms also explain the antidepressant
effects of placebos. But if depression is really a form of inflammatory disorder, caused by a pathological activation of the acute
phase response, then endorphins may be the key molecules here
too.

THE OTHER SIDE OF IMMUNITY

It may sound rather counter-intuitive to suggest that placebos work by suppressing immune activity. After all, aren't placebos supposed to make us better? There is, in fact, no contradiction here. Although the function of the immune system is to protect us from bodily damage, there are two ways in which suppressing it can be a good thing. Firstly, many aspects of immune activity, especially those involved in the acute phase response, protect us by making us *feel* bad. By suppressing these aspects of immune functioning, the placebo response can actually make us feel better. Of course, if the bad feelings are actually good for us, placebos might in fact be dangerous. They might make us feel better, but in doing so they might remove some of our vital defences against infection and injury.

This is certainly possible. Nevertheless, there are times when the bad feelings and other symptoms that accompany the acute phase response are no longer of any use. Pain, swelling and fever can all outlive their usefulness, and this indeed is what seems to happen in the chronic inflammatory disorders such as arthritis and, perhaps, depression. As its name suggests, the acute phase response was designed to be a relatively brief process. Its role in mammals like ourselves, in fact, is merely to hold the fort until another kind of immune activity kicks in. This second type of immune activity is known as acquired immunity.

There are many ways of dividing up the various elements of the immune system, but perhaps the most important is the distinction between the innate immune system and the acquired immune system. The job of both is to distinguish between self and non-self, but the innate immune system is very ancient, and is found in all animals, including insects and molluscs, whereas the acquired immune system evolved much later and is found only in vertebrates, such as fish, birds and mammals. Unlike the acquired immune system, which can recognise and remember the unique details of each species of bacterium it encounters, the innate immune system works by recognising a few simple characteristics that many bacteria have in common. In the early years of immunology, most research concentrated on unravelling the mechanisms of acquired immunity, which proved to be devilishly complex. The innate immune response was deemed to be a primitive evolutionary leftover, superseded by the sophisticated machinery of the T-cells, B-cells and memory cells that target particular invaders and not others.

Since the late 1990s, however, immunologists have become increasingly aware of the important role that the innate immune response continues to play in defending even the higher animals from infection and injury.[16] The acquired immune response may well be more effective in fighting infection, but it has one major defect – it is incredibly slow. In fact, it takes several days before an effective acquired response can be mounted against a particular pathogen, during which time the invading bacterium or virus will have multiplied many times over, gaining ever more of a foothold in the body. The innate immune response, on the other hand, can be activated within minutes of infection, and plays a vital role keeping the invaders at bay until the acquired response can eventually launch its devastating counter-attack. Were it not for the ability of the innate immune response to 'hold the fort' in this way, the acquired response might never get a chance to act; the organism might already be dead, overwhelmed by the pathogen before a proper counter-attack was even launched.

The activation of the innate immune response in the early stages of infection or injury is simply another name for the acute phase response. The acute phase response, as we have seen, takes only minutes to activate, producing pain, swelling and the various components of sickness behaviour, which can last for several days, long enough for the acquired immune system to build up its forces. Eventually, the acquired immune system is ready to take over, and the acute phase response can be turned off. Sometimes, however, for various reasons that remain obscure, the normal control mechanism that turns off the acute phase response malfunctions, and the pain, inflammation and sickness behaviour persist. The acute phase, so to speak, is no longer acute; it has become chronic. As already noted, this is what happens in certain kinds of inflammatory disorder, of which depression may be one. In this case, the placebo response would be unambiguously beneficial. It would not simply make you *feel* better; it would actually cure the underlying pathology, by turning off the inflammatory response that has managed to persist beyond the acute period for which it was designed.

Not all inflammatory disorders result from a failure to turn off the acute phase response. Some, such as juvenile onset (type 1) diabetes and asthma, are due to various components of the acquired immune system rather than the innate immune system. The fact that there are various kinds of inflammation, driven by different types of immune activity, might explain why placebos are effective against certain kinds of inflammatory disorder but not others. The fact that placebos can alleviate postoperative swelling and depression, but not juvenile onset diabetes or asthma, suggests that they can only suppress the kind of inflammation produced by the innate immune system but not the various types generated by the acquired immune system.

Placebos may also alleviate inflammation by a mechanism that has little to do with any immune activity, whether innate or acquired. There is a kind of inflammation known as neurogenic inflammation, in which the sensory nerves directly cause the blood vessels to dilate and become more permeable.[17] This helps the immune cells flow out of the blood vessels into the surrounding tissue, but it is not in itself, strictly speaking, an immune reaction. Administration of local painkillers can block neurogenic inflammation, and it is likely that the body's own painkillers – endorphins – have the same effect. The power of placebos to reduce local inflammation may therefore result from the reversal of the neurogenic component of the inflammatory process – by reducing the local blood flow and permeability of blood vessels – rather than from the inhibition of the acute phase response.

Since there is no direct evidence that endorphins play any role at all in suppressing the acute phase response, and since it is known that endorphins may block inflammation by direct effects on the sensory nerves, the hypothesis that placebos work by suppressing the acute phase response must be regarded, for the time being, as merely speculative. The research in this area is still in its infancy, but it is surely worth exploring the idea further in view of the impressive coincidence between the range of placebo-responsive conditions and the phenomena involved in the acute phase.

CHECKS AND BALANCES

If placebos really do work by suppressing the acute phase response, they would be genuinely beneficial for those inflammatory disorders that result from a failure to terminate this response. But what about normal cases of early inflammation? Surely, then, it would be risky to suppress the acute phase response before the acquired immune system has had time to get going? As already noted, the innate immune system plays a vital role in keeping infectious agents at bay while the acquired immune system builds up enough strength to fight the final battle. If the acute phase response was suppressed too quickly, before the acquired response was fully primed, this might give the invading pathogens a useful time-window in which they could flourish unchecked by either the innate or the acquired immune system.

Perhaps. We have not taken into account, however, the fact that innate immunity and acquired immunity are, to some extent, antagonistic. When bacteria have entered the body, the macrophages that are part of the innate immune system start to attack them by secreting nitric oxide, which slows down the rate at which bacteria divide. Unfortunately, the nitric oxide also slows down the division of T-cells and B-cells, which form the backbone of the acquired immune response. The acute phase response not only holds the fort while the acquired response builds itself up; it also delays the arrival of the acquired immune response.

The extra delay caused to the acquired immune response by the secretion of nitric oxide is not in itself adaptive, but it is a price worth paying to keep the bacteria at bay in the early stages of infection. The dangers of allowing the bacteria to get too much of a head start before the acquired immune system can mount its counter-attack must be great, especially if the energy and resources required by the acquired immune system are in short supply. If, however, there were some way for an organism to detect that the acquired immune system would have lots of support, then it might be beneficial to suppress the innate immune response rather earlier than if the support were not there. This, in fact, may be why the placebo response evolved. That, however, is another story, and must wait for a later chapter.

EXPLAINING THE LIMITS OF THE PLACEBO RESPONSE

If placebos really work by suppressing the acute phase, this would certainly explain why the placebo response cannot relieve other symptoms as effectively as it relieves pain, inflammation and depression. As a general rule, we would not expect placebos to benefit patients suffering from conditions that do not involve the activation of the acute phase response. And, since most medical conditions are not particularly closely connected with the acute phase response, it follows that the range of placebo-responsive conditions is very limited.

Bacterial and viral infections, for example, have not been shown to respond to placebos. This is not surprising, given that the fight against most infectious agents is largely conducted by the acquired immune system rather than the innate immune system. In theory placebos could, by suppressing the acute phase response, speed up the activation of the acquired immune response, but this has never been demonstrated in practice.

Besides, if the innate immune response were suppressed too early, before the acquired immune response had been primed, the body would be left without either kind of defence, and the infectious agent could proliferate unchecked. It does not seem likely, therefore, that placebos will ever prove to be of great use in treating infections.

Likewise, most forms of chronic degenerative disease are also probably beyond the reach of placebos. These diseases involve the gradual deterioration and loss of function of the cells of an organ or tissue, often caused by the accumulation of deposits of calcium salts, fat or fibrous tissue. Alzheimer's disease, for example, seems to involve the accumulation of excess amyloid protein in certain parts of the brain. This gradual build-up of unwanted material has little to do with the innate immune system, so there is scant reason to expect that suppressing the acute phase response will do much for helping patients with these diseases. There does, however, appear to be at least one interesting exception to this general rule. Although the evidence is not terribly strong, one or two studies have suggested that Parkinson's disease may respond to placebos. Parkinson's disease is a chronic degenerative disorder that involves a deficiency of dopamine in a region of the brain known as the basal ganglia. Like other degenerative conditions, Parkinson's disease has little to do with the acute phase response, and so it would seem to pose a problem for the theory proposed in this chapter. As we will see in Chapter Four, however, there is a good reason why this particular condition may be an exception to the general rule that placebo-responsive conditions involve the activation of the acute phase response.

Finally, of course, the various forms of cancer have nothing to do with the acute phase response, so it is hardly surprising that they do not seem to respond to placebos either. The immune system does contain cells that can attack tumours. Natural killer cells are a type of white blood cell that can detect and destroy cancerous cells. They have, at least, been observed to do so in experiments when natural killer cells extracted from someone's body have been introduced into cultures of cancer cells grown in a petri dish. Their role in fighting cancer inside the body, however, is much less clear. According to the intuitively appealing theory of 'immune surveillance', natural killer cells patrol the body looking for nascent tumours and wiping them out before they can spread to other areas of the body. Although there is some evidence to support this view, it is far from proven. Even if it does turn out to be right, it would not license talk about the immune system 'curing' cancer. It would probably be more accurate to describe the role of the immune system in fighting cancer as one of prevention rather than cure.

If natural killer cells really can destroy tumours, they can only do so long before the cancer has spread to other parts of the body, when the tumour is very small. A tumour that has become large enough to be detected by doctors must thus have escaped immune surveillance. Having got past the natural killer cells so far, it is unlikely to be picked up by them later on. By the time someone is diagnosed as suffering from cancer, therefore, it is probably too late for the immune system to do anything. Its role in protecting the body from cancer is limited to destroying tumours in their earliest stages. Furthermore, it seems that the immune system can only defend the body against a limited range of cancers. Malignant melanoma and renal cell carcinoma, for example, seem to be much more susceptible to immune defences than other kinds of cancer.

It might be thought that, since the mind can make us ill, it can also make us well again. The case of cancer shows this argument to be badly flawed. Suppose, for example, that people with depression have a slightly higher risk of getting cancer. In fact, the evidence for this link is far from conclusive. The point is that, even if the link between depression and cancer was well established, we could not infer from this that cancer can be *cured* by *optimism*. The immune system can help prevent certain kinds of cancer from developing, so it would not be surprising if those with depression, which is linked with immune dysregulation, turn out to have an increased risk of those types of cancer.

If, however, the immune system does not destroy a tumour in its early stages, it will almost certainly be incapable of destroying it later on, even if boosted by a positive mental attitude. It is not surprising, then, that we do not have any good evidence that placebos can cure cancer. By the time someone knows they have cancer, it is probably beyond the power of the immune system to reverse it.

NAUSEA, FEVER AND LETHARGY

One of the marks of a good scientific theory is that it should not only explain the data already at hand, but make accurate predictions about new facts that have not yet been discovered. Does the theory proposed here, linking the placebo effect to the suppression of the acute phase response, meet this condition? Certainly it explains the pattern in the data we examined in Chapter Two, as all the conditions listed there are related to activation of the acute phase response. It also explains why certain diseases such as cancer are beyond the power of the placebo. But what about other conditions for which there is no evidence yet either way? Are there some further medical problems which the theory predicts might be susceptible to placebos? If there are, we could put the theory to the test by seeing whether or not these conditions do, in fact, respond to placebos.

As we have already seen, nausea, fever and lethargy are all aspects of the acute phase response. If placebos work by suppressing the acute phase response, then these conditions should also be placebo-responsive. So far there is little evidence either way on this question, but there are nonetheless some tantalising hints that placebos can indeed stop you feeling sick. In one study, scientists observed stomach movements in a group of pregnant women who suffered from extreme morning sickness. The women were told that they would be given a powerful drug to cure the nausea, but the drug they actually received was, in fact, known to produce nausea rather than relieve it.

Not only did the women feel less sick after the injection, but their stomachs showed an objective decrease in the type of movement associated with nausea. In this case, the placebo effect had actually *reversed* the action of a powerful drug.[18]

When it comes to the question of whether placebos can affect fever and lethargy, not even this scant level of data is available yet. It would, however, be easy to set up experiments to test the hypothesis that these conditions too are placebo-responsive. It should be clear by now what sort of experiment would be needed. A randomised clinical trial involving patients with fever or chronic fatigue, in which half of the participants received placebos and half received no treatment at all, would be ideal, although it might be difficult to get approval for such a trial from an ethics committee. Other designs might be possible, such as giving febrile patients antipyretic drugs in different-coloured tablets, much as the team from Newcastle did with the experiment on anxiety mentioned earlier. If fever responded better to tablets of one colour rather than another, this would be evidence of a placebo effect, since the only way that tablet colour could affect fever would be by way of affecting the patient's mind.

HEART DISEASE REVISITED

One further thought is that the theory proposed in this chapter might throw some light on the mysterious links between placebos and heart disease. As we saw in Chapter Two, doctors investigating the operation of internal mammary ligation in the late 1950s found that a placebo operation was just as effective as the real thing. Patients with angina who received a sham operation, in which the surgeon cut into the chest and then stitched it back up again but without cutting off the arteries, showed the same level of improvement as those whose arteries were ligated. At the time, this was taken as proof that the operation was useless, since it was shown to be no better than a placebo. However, as we have already noted, the fact that the real operation was no better than a placebo does not mean it was necessarily 'useless'. If angina was placebo-responsive, a placebo would certainly be better than nothing. To find out whether angina really is placebo-responsive, of course, we would have to compare the improvement shown by those receiving the sham operation with those who receive no operation at all. This has not been done, but the success rates of both operations – the real one and the sham – were high enough to suggest that the placebo did produce real benefits. Not only did those receiving the operations feel less pain as a result, but they also improved on some objective measures, such as being able to walk longer distances and consuming fewer drugs.

In Chapter Two I suggested that these objective improvements might be due simply to the reduction in pain caused by the placebo. As has been noted, a person who feels less pain when walking can walk further, and will feel less of a need to take drugs. There is, though, another possibility. The reason that the arteries get blocked in heart disease is that certain blood cells known as platelets become too sticky, and clog up the coronary arteries. Platelets are the smallest of human blood cells, and usually circulate freely, but when a blood vessel is damaged it releases substances which cause the platelets to become sticky. This allows the platelets to adhere to the broken blood vessel and stop the injured person from bleeding to death. The substances that cause platelets to become sticky are yet another component of the acute phase response that enables us to respond to bodily damage.

Perhaps heart disease, then, is also caused by an over-active acute phase response. Certainly, various other conditions that involve the acute phase response are among the risk factors for heart disease. It is well known, for example, that anxiety and stress increase the risk of heart disease. Less well known, but equally suggestive, is the fact that people who suffer from severe depression are up to four times more likely to die from heart disease caused by obstructed blood flow than people who are not depressed – even when other risk factors such as smoking and high cholesterol are taken into account.[19] In fact, depression is a greater risk factor for heart disease than smoking.

Since anxiety and depression are now thought to involve the activation of the acute phase response, the link between these conditions and heart disease may lie in the increased levels of sticky platelets triggered by the inflammatory response. In 1996, Dominique Musselman of Emory University in Altlanta, Georgia, produced some initial support for this idea. She and her colleagues took blood samples from both depressed and healthy volunteers, and found that the numbers of sticky platelets were 41 per cent higher in depressed people. A few years later, the team showed that antidepressant drugs can reduce the numbers of sticky platelets in the blood of depressed patients.[20]

It is possible, then, that placebos might decrease the risk of heart disease in the same way that they help to alleviate anxiety and depression – by suppressing the acute phase response. In that case, it would be understandable why people with angina who reported improvement after the placebo operation did not show the objective signs of recovery the doctors had hoped for – post mortems revealed that no new arteries had sprouted. Perhaps the doctors were simply looking for the wrong *kind* of objective improvement. If placebos really can help those suffering from heart disease, they might do so by reducing the number of sticky platelets, not by causing new blood vessels to appear. Once again, it seems that the key to understanding the placebo response lies in understanding how the mind can suppress the acute phase response. The next step is to discover what mental process is involved. This is the subject of the next chapter.

Chapter 4

THE BELIEF EFFECT

The placebo response is beginning to look less mysterious. The range of placebo-responsive conditions, which seemed a motley collection at first sight, turns out to have an underlying logic, based in the acute phase response. The principal mechanism involved in the placebo response – the release of endogenous opiates – seems to work by suppressing the acute phase response. But this still leaves many questions unanswered. In particular, the various triggers that set the mechanism into action remain mysterious. When, and in response to what, do people suppress the acute phase response?

TRACING THE CHAIN BACK TO THE BRAIN

The range of things that are capable of triggering the placebo response is, at first sight, as baffling and bizarre as the list of placebo-responsive conditions must appear to someone unfamiliar with the acute phase response. The typical image that comes into mind when the word 'placebo' is mentioned may be a sugar pill, or perhaps some other physical substance such as an injection of saline solution; but, as will already be clear, 'sham' surgical operations can also trigger placebo responses. Later, we will examine evidence that psychotherapy, acupuncture and homeopathy can also elicit placebo responses.

The key to triggering the placebo response must be something that all these different kinds of intervention have in common. Yet it must also be something that is sometimes absent from each of these interventions, for there is no guarantee that any one of these various processes will produce a placebo response every time. The secret ingredient that triggers the placebo response must be something that can accompany sugar pills, sham surgery and psychotherapy in some contexts, but can be absent from them in others.

There is, at present, no scientific consensus as to exactly what this secret ingredient is, beyond the simple observation that it must be some process or event in the brain. The release of endorphins in the body is not by itself a full-fledged placebo response, unless it is set in motion by a particular kind of neural process. If, therefore, the local release of endorphins could be stimulated by the topical injection of a new drug, this might well result in the suppression of the acute phase response, but it would not constitute a placebo response. The placebo response does not denote a single chemical event, but a chain of such events. The chain ends in the local release of endorphins – and perhaps of other chemicals too – in the body; but it begins with a process in the brain.

So far, so good. Nobody doubts that the placebo response begins with some neural process. The disagreements start when one tries to say exactly which *kind* of neural process is involved. Part of the problem is that scientists disagree about the best way to describe *any* process in the brain. Some psychologists prefer to use mentalistic terms such as 'belief', 'desire' and 'emotion', while others prefer to avoid this kind of language and speak instead about observable behaviour. Neuroscientists do neither, focusing instead on descriptions couched in anatomical, chemical and cellular terms. For some kinds of neural process, these different approaches may co-exist peacefully, and may even be mutually inter-translatable. With most brain processes, however, this goal of conceptual integration is still a long a way off in practice. For the time being, therefore, it looks as if different kinds of neural phenomena will require different types of description.

DOPAMINE AND PARKINSON'S DISEASE

Most attempts to characterise the neural process that initiates the placebo response have so far been couched in psychological language of one kind or another. This is probably because nobody yet has much of a clue about how to describe the process in anatomical or chemical terms. Anatomically at least, the neural basis of the placebo is a mystery. Nobody knows where in the brain the key events take place that trigger the local release of endorphins in the body. Indeed, it may be a mistake to look for such a region. For a long time, many neuroscientists assumed that there would be a dedicated 'pain-centre' in the brain, but it is now known that there is no such thing; pain signals are processed by a wide range of structures dotted all over the brain. Given the close links between pain and other aspects of the acute phase response, and the complex range of stimuli that can trigger the suppression of this response, it seems likely that the neural events underlying the placebo response will be widely distributed across many different tracts of neural tissue.

Chemically speaking, things are not much clearer, although some tantalising clues have recently begun to emerge. In August 2001, scientists at the University of British Columbia in Vancouver announced that they had discovered a mechanism for the placebo effect in Parkinson's disease.[1] The commonest symptom of Parkinson's disease is a tremor in one or more limbs. As was noted in Chapter Three, the central defect in Parkinson's disease seems to be a decline in the amount of dopamine in the basal ganglia. The Canadian scientists took six patients with Parkinson's disease and scanned their brains to compare their response to an active drug (apomorphine injections) and a placebo (saline injections) − which were given in double-blind fashion. They found that, compared to a normal baseline of no treatment, there was a significant increase in levels of dopamine in the basal ganglia in response to both the active drug *and* the placebo.

It must be stressed that, although the Canadian study did find evidence that placebos could produce brief increases in the amount of dopamine in the brains of patients with Parkinson's disease, this does not necessarily mean that Parkinson's disease is placebo-responsive. There is a world of difference between triggering a brief surge of dopamine and producing the long-lasting restoration of dopamine levels that would be necessary to produce anything like a cure. Nevertheless, even if placebos cannot really cure Parkinson's disease in any meaningful sense of the term, the Canadian study suggests that they might at least be capable of producing some short-term relief. Even this modest result might seem to count against the theory proposed in the previous chapter, that all the placebo-responsive conditions involve the activation of the acute phase response, for Parkinson's disease does not appear to be related to the acute phase response.

The apparent contradiction dissolves when one remembers that the placebo response is typically a chain of events that begins in the brain and ends in the local release of endorphins at some point in the body. In most of the placebo-responsive conditions described in Chapter Two, it is the final event in this chain that produces the relief. The local release of endorphins in the mouth, for example, reduces postoperative dental pain and swelling in that area. In the case of Parkinson's disease, however, it may be the first event in the chain that counts. The neural event which normally produces a placebo response only by initiating a cascade of other chemical reactions may, in this case, be sufficient by itself to bring some relief. This is because the neural event at the root of the placebo response may be characterised, in chemical terms, by the release of dopamine, which just happens to be what those with Parkinson's disease need.

THE PSYCHOLOGICAL LEVEL OF DESCRIPTION

Our ability to describe the neural event that initiates the typical placebo response in anatomical or chemical terms is clearly very limited. Perhaps we can make more progress by using a different idiom – that of psychology. Some day, we may hope, the two approaches may come together, and we may be able to jump freely back and forth between the language of the neuroscientist and that of the psychologist. It will not matter whether we talk about an 'expectation' or a 'surge of dopamine' – they will mean the same thing. Some doubt that this scientific dream will ever become reality; and even if it does it is surely a long way off. For the time being, we must be content to pursue both types of enquiry on their own terms.

Among those who prefer to describe the neural events underlying the placebo response in psychological terms, each theorist has his own preferred terminology. Some place all the emphasis on a learning process known as conditioning. Others prefer to talk about 'expectancies'. Both of these words are already established terms of art in psychology, and those who conceive of the placebo response in these terms are simply extending existing psychological theories. Other researchers argue that we need a whole new vocabulary. For example, Daniel Moerman, an anthropologist at the University of Michigan at Dearborn, has argued that we should reconceptualise the placebo effect in terms of what he calls 'the meaning response', which he defines as the physiological or psychological effects of meaning in the treatment of illness.

My proposal is much simpler. It strikes me that we do not need any complex technical terms, either old or new, to describe the psychological ingredient in the placebo response. We already have a very ordinary, very serviceable word that encompasses all the partial insights expressed in the various technical terms just listed – *belief*. Belief is the secret ingredient in the placebo response.

REAL DRUGS AND HORSESHOES

When the famous physicist Nils Bohr was visited by a colleague one day, the visitor was shocked to observe a good-luck horseshoe hanging on the wall. 'Surely you are not superstitious?' he exclaimed. 'Oh no,' replied Bohr, 'but I am told it works whether you believe in it or not.' Bohr was joking; he knew that horseshoes do not bring good luck, even if you *do* believe in them. Drugs like etorphine, which is ten thousand times more powerful than morphine, and is used in darts by wildlife experts to immobilise big game, are another matter; they will work even if you *don't* believe in them. Most things are like real drugs and horseshoes: they either work or they don't work, and your beliefs have no bearing on the matter.

Placebos are unusual in this respect. Unlike real drugs, placebos will not help you unless you *believe* they will. Taking a sugar pill, for example, will not relieve your pain if you do not believe it to be a painkiller. The causal sequence in a typical placebo effect, then, is as follows. First, you are given a sugar pill. This causes you to acquire a certain kind of belief, and this belief then leads to the release of the endorphins that alleviate your pain.

Clearly, not every kind of belief will trigger a placebo response. If you have a headache and your doctor gives you a sugar pill, telling you that it is just a sugar pill, you may not experience any relief from your pain. But then again, you may think that your doctor is lying, and that he is in fact secretly giving you a powerful painkiller. Everything depends on what you happen to believe about the particular situation you find yourself in. So, what is it that distinguishes those beliefs that trigger the placebo response from those that do not?

The most scientific way to answer this question would be to collect a sample of beliefs that have triggered placebo responses and look for some factor, or perhaps some set of factors, that they have in common. Unfortunately, that is easier said than done. There is no foolproof method of identifying the beliefs that people hold, let alone the particular beliefs that they entertain just before their endorphins are released.

You might think that you could simply ask people what they believe, but in fact this simple idea turns out to be very problematic. For a start, people sometimes lie, so we cannot assume that what they say accurately reflects what they believe. More worrying is the possibility that people may not even know what they believe. So, even if we could be sure that someone was not lying, we might still doubt whether his reports about his own beliefs were accurate.

SAYING IS BELIEVING

Many people baulk at the idea that someone can be mistaken about his or her own beliefs. They feel that a believer must be the final authority on what his or her beliefs are. Philosophers, with their fondness for technical terms, refer to this notion as the 'assent theory of belief'.[2] According to the assent theory, a person believes whatever he honestly *says* he believes. So, by definition, nobody could ever be mistaken about his own beliefs. The philosopher Bertrand Russell held something like this view, although he placed less emphasis on the external act of reporting one's beliefs, and focused instead on internal feelings. According to Russell, the difference between a statement that someone believes and a statement that he does not believe is that in the former case, whenever the statement pops up in the mind, it occurs with a 'feeling of assent'.[3]

Despite their attractive simplicity, the various versions of the assent theory of belief all have a fatal flaw: they rob the notion of belief of any scientific value, reducing it to a completely arbitrary and chaotic affair. People often say one thing, and do another. One person says he believes in God, but never does anything even vaguely religious. Another sincerely denies that she believes in ghosts, yet shivers when told her house is haunted. If each individual really were the ultimate authority on what his or her beliefs are, we would have to accept that most people are hypocrites. Not only that, but we would also have to give up the idea that people's actions can be explained, and often predicted, by referring to their beliefs.

This last point is important, for it is such a common practice. Explaining and predicting what people will do by citing their beliefs is something we all engage in all the time. If you want to explain why John took his umbrella when he went out this morning, the chances are you will say it was because he believed it was going to rain. Conversely, if you think that John believes it is going to rain, you may predict that he will take his umbrella when he leaves the house. And, on the whole, this strategy works. Yet it is hard to see how it *could* work unless there were some fairly reliable relationship between a person's beliefs and his actions. If most people were hypocrites, we could neither explain nor predict their actions on the basis of their beliefs, since there would be no reliable link between action and belief. Since we often *can* explain and predict what people will do by referring to what they believe, it follows that people cannot be such radical hypocrites as the assent theory seems to imply. So the assent theory must be wrong.

The upshot of this is that people can, in fact, be mistaken about their own beliefs. If there is a mismatch between what someone does and what he says he believes, it could be because he is lying, or perhaps he really is being hypocritical on this occasion – but it is always possible that the person concerned is simply unaware of what his true beliefs are on this particular matter. Once you admit that such a situation is possible, it becomes much harder to find out what people do in fact believe. Simply asking someone what he believes is not good enough; you must examine what he does as well. We might call this the indirect theory of belief. Beliefs are brain processes which cannot be observed directly, but whose existence can usually be reliably inferred from a person's behaviour – which includes, but is not limited to, his verbal behaviour.

One advantage of the indirect theory of belief is that it allows us to make sense of the idea that certain non-human animals have beliefs. On the assent theory of belief, of course, cats and dogs cannot have beliefs, for the simple reason that they cannot speak or otherwise give their assent to verbal propositions. I count this as another mark against the assent theory, as it strikes me as terribly anthropocentric to deny that many other higher mammals, at least, can have beliefs. When I observe my cat lurking for hours outside the door to my girlfriend's study, in which she keeps two pet rats in a cage by her desk, I have no hesitation in explaining this behaviour by reference to the cat's beliefs. My cat simply would not waste his time lying in wait by that door unless he believed that a couple of juicy rodents were frolicking behind it.

RECONSTRUCTING BELIEFS

Reconstructing what someone (or some animal) believes on the basis of his (or its) actions is something we do all the time. Suppose a ladder is propped up against a wall, and a man walking along next to the wall makes a detour around the ladder. It is a fair bet that the man believes there was a good chance that something nasty would have happened to him if he had not made the detour. The details may not be clear – perhaps the man is superstitious, or perhaps he simply worries about ladders falling on top of him – but the general outline of the belief is obvious.

At other times, it may be much harder to reconstruct the underlying beliefs, and even in simple cases a certain amount of interpretation and guesswork is inevitable. And, to many people, interpretation and guesswork don't seem very scientific. For a large part of the twentieth century, this worried some psychologists so much that they tried to dispense with the concept of belief altogether. The behaviourist movement, as it became known, attempted to put psychology on a much more scientific footing by focusing exclusively on processes that were directly observable, such as bodily movements. Unobservable entities such as beliefs, desires and other 'mental' phenomena were dismissed altogether from the realm of psychological theory.

Behaviourism is now largely out of fashion, having been usurped by another movement known as cognitivism. In the 1960s, Noam Chomsky, George Miller, Herbert Simon and other luminaries restored scientific respectability to mental processes by comparing them to the operations of a computer. The behaviourist suspicion that 'thinking' was unobservable and therefore not a proper subject for scientific investigation lost its force when it became possible for the flow of information inside computers – and, by analogy, the flow of information inside the human brain – to be described in detail, step by step. After four bizarre decades in which many psychologists had turned their backs on the mind, it was finally legitimate to talk about thoughts and beliefs again.

Besides, the fact that it can require a certain amount of interpretation and guesswork to discover what someone believes does not mean that belief is an unscientific concept. Interpretation and guesswork are involved in almost every field of scientific endeavour, including some of the most 'scientific' sciences of all, such as particle physics. Science is different from gambling, not because it involves no guesswork at all, but because it involves *good* guesswork, carefully constrained by coherent and well-tested theories.

THE BELIEF EFFECT

Bearing in mind the preceding caveats about guesswork and interpretation, then, let us proceed to reconstruct, as best we can, the essential features of the kinds of belief that trigger placebo responses.

One crucial factor seems to be the idea that some medical intervention is taking place. Simply believing that one will get better is not enough to trigger the placebo response. If it was, one would expect the placebo response to be triggered by many other circumstances besides the provision of medical help. One must believe, rather, that one has been given some powerful medicine, or other kind of treatment. Clearly, the kinds of things that will activate this belief will differ widely from culture to culture. Although medicine is a universal human practice – healers are a feature of every society known to anthropologists – the precise details of healing practices vary enormously. The symbols that identify medical contexts in the Western world – white coats, stethoscopes and so on – are quite different from those that identify a medical situation in, say, an African tribe. If someone from a remote, preliterate culture suddenly found himself transported to a modern Western hospital, and was injected with a solution of saline, he might not recognise this procedure as a medical one. In that case, the saline injection could not produce a placebo response, since it would not induce the kind of belief that is necessary to trigger such a response – the belief that one has received a powerful medical treatment.

It is not sufficient, of course, to believe that a medical intervention is taking place. One must also believe that the medical procedure is powerful. In other words, one must believe that it *works*. A Western anthropologist who can recognise the symbols of an African tribal healing ceremony will not experience a placebo response if the village shaman attempts to cure him of some ailment – unless, that is, the anthropologist comes to believe that African tribal medicine works.

Only if you believe that a medical intervention is taking place, and that it works for the condition you are suffering from, will the placebo response be activated. This does not mean that your condition will necessarily be cured. Even if the placebo response is activated, it will not have any effect on your health unless you happen to be suffering from a placebo-responsive condition.

If this theory is correct, it should be possible to induce the placebo effect without actually giving people a placebo. Wake someone up after an operation and tell him he has just been given a powerful painkiller and – providing he believes you – he should feel less pain, even if he has received nothing, not even a sugar pill. This suggests that it is somewhat misleading to talk about the *placebo* effect. Such talk obscures the fact that the effect must be due not to the placebo itself, but to the *beliefs* of the person who is taking it. Perhaps we should speak, instead, of the 'belief effect'.

Even this phrase is ambiguous, since beliefs can have various kinds of effect. When it comes to our health, two are particularly relevant. First, beliefs can make us better by causing us to take actions such as going to the doctor or consuming cough mixture. Second, beliefs can affect the immune system directly. The belief effect refers exclusively to the second pathway.

Everything we have said so far about the placebo effect could be rephrased in terms of the belief effect. The belief effect is powerful, but not omnipotent. Mere beliefs are sufficient to relieve pain, reduce inflammation and alleviate depression and anxiety, but they cannot by themselves cure cancer or schizophrenia. The reason for these limits should now be clear. It is largely beyond the power of the immune system to cure cancer and schizophrenia, so no amount of belief will help these conditions either. On the other hand, pain, inflammation and depression all involve aspects of the immune system – and, moreover, these aspects of the immune system are susceptible to psychological input. They can, in other words, be triggered by relevant beliefs.

TESTING THE BELIEF THEORY

If the placebo effect is really the belief effect – if, in other words, belief is the crucial psychological trigger that sets off the placebo response – then we should be able to influence the degree to which someone experiences placebo response by manipulating his beliefs. In order to do *that*, of course, we need to know what sort of things affect people's beliefs. Two obvious candidates are experience and verbal information imparted by an authority. In the 1990s, a series of fascinating experiments was performed to investigate how placebo responses could be altered by manipulating these two sources of belief.

The ways that one's own experience of medication can influence the placebo response have been investigated by looking at conditioning. Conditioning is a very general kind of learning process in which one stimulus is substituted for another. The classic example is Pavlov's dogs. When the famous Russian psychologist Ivan Pavlov noticed that hungry dogs salivated profusely not only at the sight of food, but also of the attendant who fed them, he decided to investigate the phenomenon experimentally. By consistently exposing his dogs to various stimuli – a bell, a metronome, a flashing light – just before feeding them, Pavlov trained his dogs to salivate at things that would not normally trigger such a response. Shortly after Pavlov's pioneering work, other Russian scientists discovered that the immune system could also be conditioned. When guinea pigs were repeatedly exposed to a neutral stimulus such as gentle scratching just before being injected with a substance that triggered an inflammatory response, their immune systems learned the association between scratching and inflammation, so that eventually gentle scratching on its own was enough to provoke swelling and redness.[4]

In the official terminology, an 'unconditioned stimulus' (the sight of the meat for Pavlov's dogs), which leads naturally to an 'unconditioned response' (salivating at the sight of the meat), is repeatedly paired with a 'conditioned stimulus' (the sound of a bell, for example). Eventually, the dogs learn the 'conditioned response' of salivating at the sound of the bell.

The placebo effect, it has been claimed, works in exactly the same way.[5] The unconditioned stimulus is a real drug, or some other kind of medical treatment that works even if you have never tried it before, and the unconditioned response is the improvement that ensues after receiving this treatment. The conditioned stimuli are all the things that are repeatedly paired with taking the drug. Suppose, for example, you notice that the pill is always pink and round, and is always prescribed by a man in a white coat. After being prescribed this pill several times, you will come to associate these other conditions with the feeling of getting better. Then, if the doctor gives you a pink pill with no medication in it, you will respond by getting better, just as Pavlov's dogs salivated in response to a bell that was not accompanied by food.

Since we know that the immune system can be conditioned

just like salivation and other biological responses, the conditioning theory of placebos is certainly plausible. But what about the
evidence? Support for the conditioning theory is provided
by several intriguing studies conducted by the psychologist
Nicholas Voudouris and his colleagues at La Trobe University
in Australia. In one study, Voudouris prepared a fake analgesic
cream by mixing simple cold cream with linalol, which gave it
a distinct smell.[6] He told ten volunteers that the cream was a
local painkiller, and connected their arms to a special device
designed to generate pain by driving potassium ions into the
skin. At lower levels of stimulation, the machine causes a prick-
ling sensation, but when the current is turned up it produces a
severe cramp. The machine was set initially at a very low level,
and the volunteers were asked to signal when they could no
longer tolerate the pain, at which point the machine was
switched off.

After measuring initial levels of pain tolerance with and without the placebo cream applied, Voudouris proceeded to trick
the volunteers into believing that the placebo was an effective
painkiller. The volunteers underwent a series of three pain-
tolerance tests with the cream applied, then three more tests
with the cream removed. For each test, the length of time
they could withstand the pain was measured. Unknown to the
volunteers, however, the machine was turned down when the
cream was applied, so it appeared to them as if the cream really
was blocking the pain. Finally, the volunteers were given two
more tests – one with the cream applied, and one without –
during which the machine was kept at the initial level. Sure
enough, the volunteers were able to tolerate the pain much
longer when the cream was applied in the final test than when
it had been applied in the initial test. They had learned from
the apparently incontrovertible testimony of their own experience that the cream was an effective painkiller.

Or had they? Direct experience was not, in fact, the only
source of belief in operation here. Voudouris had informed the
volunteers at the start of the experiment that the cream was a

painkiller, so another source of belief – the voice of authority – was also at work. In order to control for this, Voudouris added another twist to the experiment. He took another ten volunteers and put them through the same ordeal, but with one small difference. This time, instead of turning the machine *down* when the cream was applied, he turned it up. Now the volunteers were receiving conflicting information. On the one hand, an authority had told them that the cream was a painkiller. The evidence of their senses, on the other hand, pointed in the opposite direction: the cream, it seemed, made the pain get *worse*. When the volunteers in this group were given the final test (with the machine returned to its initial level), the result was very different. Unlike the members of the first group, the amount of time these volunteers could withstand the pain with the cream applied was now less than it had been at the start of the experiment.

Voudouris concluded, not unreasonably, that when these two sources of belief – experience and verbal information imparted by an authority figure – point in opposite directions, experience wins. It was not long, though, before two psychologists at the University of Connecticut found evidence that called this conclusion into question. In 1997, Guy Montgomery and Irving Kirsch used an experimental set-up similar to that of Voudouris, but with yet another twist.[7] As before, one group was tricked into thinking that the cream was an effective painkiller, since the machine was secretly turned down when the cream was applied. Another group was *told* that the machine was being turned down when the cream was applied. It was explained to this group that the intensity of the machine would be reduced on medication trials, so that the effectiveness of the cream could be examined at lower intensities. When the volunteers were given the final test, with the machine back at the original level, the placebo effect in the first group was significantly greater than it had been at the start of the experiment. That is, the difference between the pain felt when the cream was applied and when the cream was not applied had increased. The placebo effect in the second group, however, was unchanged. The information – relayed to them verbally by the experimenter – that the machine was being turned down when the cream was applied, changed the meaning of their experience entirely. Knowing the true source of the reduction in pain, they no longer attributed it to the cream.

Taken together, these studies suggest that, when experience and verbal information point in opposite directions, it is hard to predict which will win out. In the experiment conducted by Voudouris, experience seems to trump verbal information, while in the study by Montgomery and Kirsch it is the other way around. There is no rigid hierarchy, then, governing the importance of the various sources of belief about placebos. Experience and the voice of authority may both play a part in leading us to believe that a treatment is effective, and the relative importance of each will vary from context to context, and from person to person, in ways that we cannot yet fathom.

CONDITIONING

At this point, a little digression is called for, since I have a confession to make: I have been guilty of some reinterpretation. When Voudouris, Montgomery and Kirsch published their studies, they did not report their results in quite the same terms as those used here. Instead of posing the debate in terms of the relative strength of two sources of belief – experience and verbal information – they described it instead as a clash between two theories of the placebo effect: the conditioning theory and the expectancy theory. Voudouris argued that his studies supported conditioning theory, while Montgomery and Kirsch claimed that their experiment vindicated the expectancy theory. Despite a few half-hearted caveats hidden away towards the end of their papers, both sides gave the impression that the two theories were mutually exclusive.

This is, quite simply, rubbish. In reality, there need be no antagonism between the conditioning theory of placebos and the idea that the placebo response is triggered by expectancies. Expectancies are simply beliefs about the future, and conditioning can be regarded as one way in which such beliefs are acquired. If you have heard a bell ring just before every meal, and end up salivating at the mere sound of the bell, one way of explaining this is to say that your experience of hearing bells before meals has led you to acquire a particular belief – namely that when a bell rings, food is on its way. It is this *belief*, in combination with the sound of the bell, rather than the sound of the bell on its own, that causes you to salivate.

This way of putting things is not the way in which conditioning has typically been described. For much of the twentieth century, psychologists who wrote about conditioning tended to describe it in terms of a stimulus (the sound of the bell, for example) causing a response (such as salivation) directly, without the aid of any mediating belief. This curious way of describing conditioning arose because the first psychologists who did research in this area were behaviourists. As already noted, the behaviourists rejected all talk of mental entities such as beliefs, hopes and desires, which had played the leading role in theories about human behaviour for hundreds of years. Science, they claimed, could have no truck with woolly explanations referring to such invisible processes. Instead, psychologists should refer only to observable behaviour. The laws they aimed to discover would relate stimuli to responses directly, without postulating anything so medieval as a mind in between.

Around the same time as J.B. Watson was announcing the behaviourist manifesto in America, Pavlov and his colleagues in Russia were refining the conditioning process that would give behaviourism its experimental backbone. Their success in training animals to respond in novel ways to various sights and sounds seemed to offer just what Watson needed – firm evidence that it was possible to discover lawful generalisations linking stimuli to behaviour that made no reference to intervening thoughts.

Behaviourism might now be dead, but conditioning is certainly not. As an experimental paradigm, it is still widely used by psychologists all over the world. The historical association between the theory of behaviourism and the experimental investigation of conditioning has, however, left the impression in the minds of some psychologists that, when some form of behaviour can be conditioned, it cannot involve belief. Nothing could be further from the truth. Conditioning is best seen as one source of belief – the evidence of direct experience – which may be compatible, or at variance, with other sources of belief, such as the voice of authority.

Voudouris, Montgomery and Kirsch confused matters, then, when they interpreted their studies as evidence for or against the conditioning theory of placebos. The real importance of their work lies in the light it casts on the complex ways in which people come to believe that particular kinds of treatment will be effective, sometimes putting the evidence of their senses above the voice of authority, while at other times doing completely the opposite.

THE ELUSIVE PLACEBO REACTOR

In the early days of placebo research, just after World War II, there was a general feeling among psychologists that there must be something wrong with people who were affected by placebos. True, the placebo effect itself was a blessing, allowing those who experienced it to get relief from a mere sugar pill, but all the same, the fact that some people could believe that a mere sugar pill was a painkiller surely pointed to some defect in their cognitive machinery. Something had to be wrong with their belief-forming mechanisms, it seemed, for people to be duped into adopting such obviously false beliefs, even if these beliefs had the disconcerting capacity to make themselves true by shaping reality in their own image. Perhaps it was only particularly stupid or gullible people who could be affected by placebos.

This view chimed with another common impression among

placebo researchers at the time. Until the 1990s, it was widely believed that a fixed fraction – about a third – of the population was susceptible to the placebo effect, while the rest were not. Like so many other myths surrounding the placebo response, this idea can be traced back to Beecher's influential 1955 article on 'The Powerful Placebo'.[8] Beecher, it will be recalled, had drawn on the results of fifteen earlier placebo-controlled studies to argue that placebos had powerful effects in their own right. For each study, he noted the proportion of patients in the placebo group who had improved. This, he claimed, was an accurate measure of the placebo effect. It was not, of course. As we saw in Chapter One, this figure is meaningless without a no-treatment group to compare it with, and also fails to take into account a whole range of other complicating factors, such as the number of patients in the placebo group who got worse, the possibility that some patients in the placebo group were taking other medication outside the trial, and so on. But the methodological errors do not stop there. After noting the proportion of patients in each study who had improved after taking a placebo, Beecher went on to calculate the average improvement rate by adding up these proportions and dividing them by the number of studies. The figure he arrived at was 35 per cent.

In the decades following Beecher's paper, that figure – alternatively reported as '35 per cent' or 'about a third' – was quoted and requoted by medical researchers until, by dint of repetition, it appeared to become set in stone. The idea that placebos only worked for a fixed proportion of the population made it seem as if there was some mental trait that distinguished the 'placebo reactor' from the 'non-reactor'. Various candidates were proposed, from low intelligence to neuroticism. After years of searching for the elusive trait that separated the reactors from the non-reactors, however, placebo researchers finally admitted that they had reached an impasse. Everyone, it seemed, could respond to a placebo, given the right conditions.

With hindsight, the very idea that people could be divided

into consistent placebo reactors and consistent nonreactors seems a non-starter. The placebo effect involves physiological mechanisms common to everyone, but these are only triggered when people have the right belief, and – as we have seen – the sources of evidence are highly variable in their power to induce belief. When the authors of a study published in 1995 examined five placebo-controlled trials of painkillers conducted between 1981 and 1990, they found that individual pain-relief scores of those taking placebos varied from 0 to 100 per cent.[9] That is a long way from the figure of 35 per cent that Beecher claimed to have found 'rather constantly'.

Even in Beecher's original paper, the variation was greater than his figure of 35 per cent suggested. One of the studies he cited reported that a mere 15 per cent of those in the placebo group obtained 'satisfactory relief', while another found that the same level of relief had been obtained by as many as 58 per cent of those in the placebo group. These wide variations were concealed because Beecher chose to average across the studies. Moreover, he used a kind of average (the mean) which was not suitable for the kind of data he was analysing. More recent studies have found that most people in pain only experience a mild level of relief whether given a placebo or an active drug. Since there are usually a few people, however, who experience total, or near total, pain relief, this bumps up the mean substantially. If Beecher had used a different kind of average – the median – he would not have found such a constant proportion of 'placebo reactors', and the fruitless search for the quality that distinguished this mythical group from the rest of the world might never have started.

To be fair, then, I should add a rider to my previous remarks in praise of statistical research. Statistics can deceive as well as enlighten. They need to be interpreted with care, and certainly not blindly repeated, as the '35 per cent' figure was by placebo researchers for so many years. Statistics may well be the remedy for an uncritical dependence on authority, but there is no progress if the result is merely an uncritical dependence on numbers.

THE CLINICAL CONTEXT

By the 1970s, there was a growing consensus that placebos could affect everyone. Not only did the response rate of the placebo arm vary much more than Beecher had claimed, but the placebo response could vary within the same person between one moment and the next. If the same patient might respond to one placebo but not to another, then the crucial variable could not lie in the patient's enduring personality structure, but rather must be sought in the changing features of the clinical situation.

An example of how subtle these variations can be was discovered by accident when a group of scientists in Holland were unable to replicate an experiment in immune conditioning that had previously been carried out in Germany.[10] In the first experiment, a group of German investigators gave volunteers sherbet sweets just before injecting them with adrenaline, a hormone which is known to provoke a brief increase in natural killer cell activity. After four of these sessions (once a day on four consecutive days) the volunteers were given the sherbet as usual, but were injected with saline instead of adrenaline. Sure enough, the same increase in natural killer cell activity was triggered. The immune system had learned to boost itself in response to the combination of a sweet taste and an injection – even when the injection was a placebo.

Curiously, when the group of investigators in Holland tried the same experiment, they found that the placebo produced no effect. When they injected the volunteers with saline on the fifth day, no increase in natural killer cell activity was observed. In an attempt to explain the disparity between the two studies, the researchers looked more closely at the details of each. Two interesting but subtle differences emerged. One concerned the amount of information given to the volunteers. In contrast to the German group, the researchers in Holland were required to inform the volunteers that they were being injected with adrenaline, and what side-effects might be expected. It is possible that this extra bit of information was enough to alter the way in which the Dutch subjects interpreted their experience of the training sessions, just as the volunteers in Montgomery and Kirsch's study no longer experienced any placebo effect when informed that the intensity of the pain-generating machine was being turned down. As the attention of the Dutch volunteers had been drawn to the specific side-effects of the adrenaline, they would have been much more likely to notice their absence when injected with saline, and so less likely to acquire the mistaken belief that they were being given the same substance as before.

There were also cultural differences between the participants in the two studies. For example, Dutch subjects are generally much more critical of experiments in which they participate, while the Germans were happy to volunteer for a study even though they had no idea what they would be injected with. This greater scepticism may have led the Dutch volunteers to be on the lookout for any trick that the researchers might play on them, such as substituting a dummy injection for a real one.

If such subtle differences in the experimental set-up can completely abolish the placebo effect, we should be wary about generalising from the results of experimental studies to real clinical practice. In particular, we should be alert to the many factors that make the situation of a participant in a clinical trial or an experiment rather different from that of a patient attending a doctor's clinic, or a road-accident victim receiving emergency surgery at a hospital. The requirement for informed consent means that patients participating in a clinical trial will know that they might be given a placebo rather than a real drug. They will thus be more attentive to any clues that give away the identity of their treatment. No such doubts assail the patient who visits his doctor in search of relief for his headache, which means that the placebo effect may be increased in this context. On the other hand, patients attending a clinical trial may receive much more care and attention than someone paying a brief visit to the doctor, and this may have the reverse effect, leading to greater placebo effects in clinical trials than in the GP's surgery.

Likewise, a volunteer in a pain-tolerance test knows that the pain is not indicative of serious bodily damage, and is assured that he can pull out of the experiment whenever he wants. The victim of a real accident, however, has neither of these luxuries. Beecher reported that placebos induced much greater pain relief in real clinical settings than in artificial situations, when pain was induced experimentally.

These myriad sources of variation should come as no surprise. If the placebo effect is really just the belief effect, then its magnitude should depend on the strength of one's belief in the power of the particular treatment administered. And since the number of variables that can influence the strength of a belief is virtually unlimited, so also will be the factors that determine the extent of the placebo response. Here, it seems, science must bow its head and accept that, when it comes to the laws that govern the variations observed in the placebo response, only the most vague generalisations may be discoverable.

UNCONSCIOUS COMMUNICATION

The situation becomes even more complex when it is acknowledged that the doctor may convey more information to the patient than either of them realises. In addition to the words he speaks, the doctor gives out any number of non-verbal clues as to his expectations regarding the treatment, many of which he may not be aware of giving out. Patients pick up these clues and modify their beliefs accordingly, sometimes without even knowing it.

A stunning example of how this 'unconscious communication' between doctor and patient can influence the placebo response was reported in a letter to the *Lancet* in 1985.[11] Forty-six patients who had undergone tooth extraction were asked to indicate their level of pain before being given an injection which, they were told, might contain a painkiller (fentanyl), a pain-increaser (naloxone), or a placebo (saline). If the study had been truly double-blind, the clinicians would have remained as ignorant as the patients about who was to receive which drug. However, in order to test the effect of the clinician's expectations, the experimenters divided the patients into two groups, and told the clinicians that group one would be randomly assigned either the placebo or the pain-increaser, while the other group would be randomly divided between all three treatments (placebo, pain-increaser and painkiller). When the injections had been given, the patients were asked once more to indicate their level of pain. Those in the first group who had been given a placebo reported much less pain relief than those in the second group who had received a placebo. Since the only difference between these patients lay in the clinician's knowledge of the range of possible treatments, which had not been relayed to the patients verbally, it is clear that the patients must have picked up on subtle non-verbal clues. The clinicians had unwittingly transmitted their greater confidence in the possibility of pain relief in group two, and this information had unconsciously modified the patients' own expectations.

This phenomenon is the main reason why placebo-controlled studies should be double-blind rather than simply single-blind. If the doctors know which patients in a trial are receiving a placebo and which the real drug, they may communicate this information unintentionally, even if they never actually reveal it explicitly. This is not because doctors are particularly bad at keeping secrets; unconscious, non-verbal communication is something we all do all the time, whether we like it or not. As the rarity of good poker players testifies, keeping a secret requires a discipline of which few people are capable.

BELIEF AND MAGIC

Just because science legitimises the notion of belief, and even the idea that beliefs can affect health directly, does not mean we have to accept all the claims made about the power of faith.

We should treat claims about the power of *belief* to cure cancer with just as much scepticism as stories about the anti-cancer effects of placebos. In fact, even greater scepticism is probably in order, since there are many more claims made about the power of belief alone than about the power of placebo-induced belief. A whole industry is now geared to promoting the idea that people can cure themselves of the most severe diseases simply by adopting the right beliefs. The best-selling self-help guru Louise Hay, for example, claims to have cured herself of cancer by letting go of the feelings of resentment she had been harbouring against various people. She now teaches that 'disease can be healed, if we are willing to change the way we think and believe and act'.[12] The last clause about changing the way we act is a bit of a get-out clause, since it could conceivably cover taking the right drugs, but the real emphasis is on the power of belief unaided by action. 'What you choose to think about yourself becomes true for you,' claims Hay, and 'we have unlimited choices about what we can think.'[13]

Neither of these claims is strictly true. Some thoughts are indeed self-fulfilling: the belief that a pill will reduce pain, for example, can itself cause the pill to relieve pain. But other thoughts are powerless by themselves. Despite what Hay says, nobody has ever caused a tumour to vanish overnight merely by thinking that it will. Likewise, the idea that we are completely free to choose our beliefs is sadly mistaken. Changing our minds is simply not that easy.

We can certainly choose to *say* we have changed our mind on some issue, but that is no guarantee that we have really done so. As we have already seen, people do not always know what they really believe. If it is naive to think that one cannot be mistaken about one's own beliefs, it is equally naive to think that one can change one's mind at will.

There are only a few ways in which we can acquire new beliefs or change old ones. We have already looked briefly at two of them: accepting on trust the words of someone else whom one thinks is an authority on the matter, and learning from our own personal experience. Another way is to use logic. Logic can help us deduce previously unrecognised consequences from old beliefs, or spot inconsistencies in our beliefs that cause us to reject them. None of these three ways of changing your mind is really voluntary. Despite the powerful illusion to the contrary, you never *decide* to change your mind; it changes itself in accordance with one or more of these three criteria.

This explains why we cannot induce the belief effect in ourselves merely by willpower. Louise Hay advises her followers to repeat 'positive affirmations' to themselves, in the hope that such mindless repetition will eventually ingrain the new belief by brute force, like a kind of self-hypnosis. The technique dates back to the French psychologist Emil Coué, who recommended in the early 1920s that people should look in the mirror every day and tell themselves that 'Every day, in every way, I am getting better and better.' But there is no evidence that anyone has ever succeeded in persuading themselves that a statement is true simply by repeating it.

Give someone a placebo, however, and you might very well succeed in causing him to acquire the right belief to boost the immune system. This, in fact, is why the belief effect is so intimately bound up with placebos. Administering a placebo simply happens to be a good way of inducing the beliefs that are necessary to trigger the various immune mechanisms we looked at in the last chapter. Placebos induce these beliefs by the second and third of the three routes described. Sometimes, taking a placebo causes you to believe that you will feel less pain because someone you trust — a doctor, perhaps, or a parent — *tells* you that the sugar pill, dock leaf or whatever else is in fact a powerful painkiller. At other times, your *experience* of taking little pink pills has led you to acquire the belief that such pills typically reduce pain, so when you take another one, this causes you to believe that pain relief will follow shortly. Either way, it seems, you have very little choice in coming to that very useful belief.

Chapter 5

WHY? THE EVOLUTIONARY QUESTION

The desire to take medicine is one feature which distinguishes man, the animal, from his fellow creatures.
WILLIAM OSLER, *Teaching and Thinking* (1895)

Among the many questions surrounding the placebo response, perhaps the most mysterious is why it should exist at all. This is not the sort of question that doctors are used to asking. On the whole, medicine concerns itself with the 'what' and 'how' of health and disease. Doctors are often content when they know *what* conditions a treatment works for. Medical researchers may want to go a bit further, and discover *how* it works. Rarely does anyone take the final step, and ask *why* the body is designed in such a way as to permit the drug to work. There is, however, a small but growing movement of medical scientists who claim that this final step is vital. The name of this movement is evolutionary medicine.[1]

WHY?

'Why?' may not seem like a request for an evolutionary explanation. If someone asks, for example, why the heart is designed the way it is, we can give a good enough answer by explaining that it is a pump. As soon as we understand, in other words, what the heart's *function* is – to pump blood around the body – then the layout of the various muscles and chambers makes

96

sense. The question and the answer are both perfectly intelligible without any reference to evolution. William Harvey, the seventeenth-century British physician who discovered the circulation of the blood, was able to grasp the function of the heart two centuries before Darwin proposed his theory of evolution by natural selection.

Nevertheless, there is a sense in which Harvey's ignorance of evolution did detract from his understanding of physiology. Hearts do many other things besides pumping blood around the body. They make soft beating sounds, for example, that can be detected when one presses one's ear against someone's chest, or by using a stethoscope. Yet we do not say that the function of the heart is to make these sounds. Among all the various things that hearts do, we select one particular action – that of pumping blood – and designate this as its real function. All the other things that hearts do, such as making soft noises, are regarded as mere by-products. What grounds do we have for making this distinction?

If we were able to put this question to Harvey, he would probably respond by invoking God. The reason we say that the heart's function is to pump blood, and not to make noise, is – Harvey might observe – because God designed the heart for that reason. Today, biologists invoke a rather different designer – a blind watchmaker, a process without any foresight, a purely mechanical operation: natural selection. The justification for singling the pumping of blood out from among all the various actions of the heart, and designating this as the heart's *function*, is that it is this particular action of the heart that explains why hearts helped our ancestors to survive and reproduce. Creatures whose hearts were good at pumping blood became our ancestors, and those whose hearts were not good at pumping blood did not. The noise was beside the point; those of our ancestors who had loud hearts did not leave more offspring than those who had comparatively silent hearts. Unbeknownst to Harvey, every discovery about an organ's present function is also a glimpse into the distant past.

FUNCTION OR BY-PRODUCT?

The web of chemical messengers and psychological triggers that produce the placebo response are, like the heart, the result of millions of years of evolution. And, like the heart, these complex mechanisms produce many other effects besides suppressing the acute phase response. As in the case of the heart and the action of pumping blood, we can ask whether the placebo response is the *function* of the mechanisms that produce it, or a mere by-product. Is the placebo response, in other words, like the action of pumping blood, or like the action of making soft beating sounds? Did the mechanisms that enable the placebo response to occur evolve for this very reason? Or for some other purpose?

Before attempting to answer this question, let us spell out the two possible answers in more detail. The first possibility is that the placebo response is an adaptation designed by natural selection. In other words, the mechanisms that produce the placebo response allowed those of our ancestors who possessed such mechanisms to survive and reproduce more successfully than those who lacked them. If this were the case, then the placebo response would be a true function of the mechanisms that produce it. Of course, we would have to spell out how, exactly, the evolution of the placebo response helped our ancestors to survive and reproduce more successfully. What particular advantages did the capacity to respond to placebos confer on those who possessed it?

The other possibility is that the placebo response is not a true function of the mechanisms that produce it, but a mere by-product, like the soft sounds made by the beating heart. Perhaps the mechanisms that underlie the placebo response evolved for some other reason, and it is just an accident that they also enable us to respond to placebos. Perhaps the placebo response is not advantageous. Perhaps it is even deleterious, but for various reasons has not been eliminated by natural selection. The human body is riddled with design faults which natural selection has not yet been able to eliminate. The fact that the windpipe leading from our noses to our lungs, for example, intersects with the digestive tract leading from our mouths to our stomachs, means that we are at risk of choking to death.[2] A clever designer would probably relocate the human mouth above the nose so as to avoid this risk, but that is not a viable option for natural selection. Unlike human designers, the blind watchmaker cannot solve design problems by going back to the drawing board and starting over from scratch. Each improvement must be brought about by a series of tiny steps, each of which is itself an improvement over the previous one. When the path to an improvement involves a temporary loss of function, it is beyond the reach of natural selection. As a result, some defects become 'developmentally entrenched'. They are, in the evocative words of the science writer Elaine Morgan, 'the scars of evolution', and we are stuck with them.[3]

IMMUNE CONDITIONING

In order to determine whether the placebo response is an adaptation or a by-product, it is first necessary to get some idea about when the capacity to respond to placebos first evolved. This is not an easy matter. In the absence of a time machine, biologists must resort to the indirect evidence provided by comparative studies. If we discovered, for example, that the placebo response was found only in humans, this would suggest that the capacity to respond to placebos evolved relatively late, after the human lineage had diverged from that leading to modern chimpanzees. If, on the other hand, we found that the placebo response was widespread among mammals, this would be good evidence that it evolved much earlier, no later than the time when the last common ancestor of all mammals walked the earth.

Which animals, then, other than humans, can respond to placebos? Scientists have found that many mammals seem to be subject to *something like* the placebo effect. To be specific, rats, mice, guinea pigs and dogs have all been shown to be susceptible to a phenomenon known as *immune conditioning*. Conditioning, as we saw in the last chapter, is a kind of learning in which one event comes to be associated with another. When the conditioned response is some kind of immune activity, the process is referred to as immune conditioning.

Immune conditioning was first discovered by Russian scientists in the first decades of the twentieth century, but these early studies passed largely unnoticed by Western biologists until the phenomenon was rediscovered half a century later by two American scientists. Robert Ader and Nicholas Cohen − a psychologist and an immunologist − stumbled across it almost by accident, when they investigated a form of conditioning known as learned taste aversion.[4] By repeatedly injecting rats with cyclophosphamide (a drug that induces nausea) whenever they drank sweetened water, Ader and Cohen succeeded in training the rats to avoid sweet water. Unfortunately for the poor rats, however, it seemed that their immune systems had been affected too, and they began to die in unexpectedly large numbers. Besides inducing nausea, cyclophosphamide also suppresses the immune system, so Ader and Cohen had inadvertently conditioned the rats to suppress their own immune responses whenever they drank the sweet water. In fact, the more sweet water the rats had consumed, the more likely they were to die.

Ader and Cohen decided to investigate the phenomenon further by means of similar experiments in which immune functioning was measured directly. After conditioning the rats by pairing sweet water with injections of cyclophosphamide, they injected them with sheep red blood cells, which, although harmless, provoke an antibody response. Then they gave some of the conditioned rats more sweet water but injected them with a placebo − a solution of saline − instead of cyclophosphamide. Sure enough, the rats given the placebo had a reduced antibody response to the sheep blood cells compared to rats that were not re-exposed to the sweet water. The rats had learned that injections after sweet water suppressed their immune systems, and so they responded by suppressing their immune systems themselves when faced with what they thought was the same situation again – even though it was not, in fact, exactly the same situation, since the cyclophosphamide had been replaced by saline. The rats had, so to speak, been tricked into suppressing their own immune systems.[5]

Humans, too, are susceptible to immune conditioning. The evidence for this comes not from experimental studies, as it would probably be unethical to perform such experiments on humans, but from observations of clinical situations such as the chemotherapy of cancer patients. Besides destroying cancer cells, chemotherapy has the unfortunate side-effect of destroying the body's own immune cells too, and so is not unlike cyclophosphamide in suppressing immune activity. Not surprisingly, the body resists chemotherapy, and reacts to it with feelings of nausea and consequent vomiting. In the 1980s, doctors noticed that cancer patients who had been receiving chemotherapy would start to feel nauseous and even vomit on arrival at the hospital, before they had been given that day's dose. The doctors guessed that the conditioned vomiting might also be a symptom of conditioned immunosuppression, just as in the case of Ader and Cohen's rats.

To test out this theory, one group of researchers measured various indices of immune activity in a group of women cancer patients several days before their scheduled chemotherapy session, and again in the hospital just before treatment.[6] While there was no change in some of these measures, there were significant reductions in others. The association of the hospital environment and the chemotherapy had become so ingrained that the mere sight of the place (or perhaps its smell) was enough to trigger a decrease in immune activity.

PLACEBOS FOR RATS?

It was not long before several researchers began to suggest that immune conditioning might play a part in the placebo effect. Some, indeed, argued that this was all there was to the placebo effect. An early study showing that rats could be conditioned to respond to injections of saline as if they contained a sedative, for example, announced its results under the dramatic title 'Placebo Effect in the Rat'.[7]

This, however, is to stretch language rather too far. Immune conditioning is a much broader category than the placebo response. All sorts of immune activity can be conditioned, including activation of the inflammatory response. The placebo effect, however, seems to be restricted to suppression of the inflammatory response. This, at least, was the argument in Chapter Three. So the placebo response is probably best seen as just one particular kind of immune conditioning. This is in part a semantic issue about what we *choose* to regard as examples of the placebo response, of course. However, since the phenomenon of immune conditioning is already well defined, while the placebo response is not, it would seem preferable to keep the two terms separate, rather than having two words for the same thing.

Besides, it seems that conditioning alone is not sufficient to account for all the complexities of the placebo response in humans. As we saw in the last chapter, the key factor in activating the placebo response is belief, and, in humans at least, there are other sources of belief besides the direct experience of conditioning. In particular, higher cognitive processes such as reasoning and the processing of verbal information are also involved in affecting people's responses to placebos, and sometimes these cognitive processes can override the effects of conditioning. To equate the placebo response with immune conditioning would be to dismiss these higher cognitive processes as largely irrelevant to understanding placebos. Yet, for many of those who investigate placebos, the role of higher cognitive processes is one of the most fascinating aspects of the whole topic.

Although rats and dogs are susceptible to immune conditioning, the subtleties of verbal information are lost on them, so the capacity for the full-fledged placebo response must have evolved much later than immune conditioning itself. Still, immune conditioning was almost certainly a vital precursor of the placebo effect proper. The capacity to respond to placebos may well be more than just immune conditioning, but it could not have evolved unless immune conditioning had already been in place.

Before we can ask, then, about the reasons for the evolution of the placebo response itself, we must first discover why immune conditioning evolved. Here, the same fundamental alternative we looked at earlier is also relevant. Either immune conditioning evolved by natural selection, in which case it must have conferred an evolutionary advantage on those who had it, or it is a by-product that evolved by chance.

THE EVOLUTION OF IMMUNE CONDITIONING

It is not hard to see how the capacity for immune conditioning could provide an evolutionary advantage to those animals that possess it. Immune agents such as antibodies are precious resources, and there is no point in generating them if they are going to be destroyed by an immunosuppressive drug. Any animal that could learn to suppress its own immune system when faced with a substance like cyclophosphamide would avoid wasting its resources and could, perhaps, save them for a later date. This, then, might be the reason why animals first acquired the ability to suppress their immune systems in response to sensory information.

There is, however, a problem with this theory: the immune system can be conditioned to boost itself as well as to suppress itself. Indeed, this was revealed by some of the very first experiments in immune conditioning. We have already seen how Russian scientists discovered that guinea pigs could be conditioned to associate gentle scratching and inflammation, so that eventually gentle scratching on its own was enough to provoke swelling and redness. Inflammation is, as we have seen, a symptom of immune activation, so it seems that immune enhancement can be conditioned as well as immune suppression.

Conditioned enhancement of the immune system has also been demonstrated in humans. In one study, for example, scientists compared a measure of macrophage activity in two groups of healthy volunteers. Over four weeks, the first group was given a course of oral placebos, each of which was accompanied by an injection of gamma interferon, which stimulates macrophage activity. The second group was also given the course of oral placebos, which were also paired with injections of gamma interferon to start with, but were progressively weaned off the injections so that by the last week they received only the placebo. At the end of the study, the second group had higher levels of macrophage activity than those who had received the gamma interferon all along.[8]

The fact that the immune system can be conditioned to enhance its activity as well as to suppress it is a blow for the theory that immune conditioning evolved for the purpose of preventing wastage. However, it is not necessarily a fatal one. Immune conditioning might still have evolved to prevent wastage, and the capacity for conditioning to enhance immune activity might simply be an unintended side-effect. Perhaps the physiological and neural machinery necessary for the former inevitably provides the capacity for the latter. If this were the case then immune conditioning could still have evolved to prevent wastage, provided that it tended to result, most of the time, in immunosuppression.

We are now deep in the realm of speculation, but there is some evidence that supports this view. For one thing, there is far more evidence for conditioned immunosuppression than there is for conditioned immunoenhancement. Of course, this might simply be due to the bias of the researchers themselves – more studies have set out to investigate how conditioning can suppress the immune system than to look at how it can enhance immune activity. However, the results of the studies that have tried to find evidence of conditioned immunoenhancement have been much less consistent than those that have investigated conditioned immunosuppression. In one study, for example, volunteers were conditioned to associate substances from different-coloured vials with different immune responses.[9] At monthly intervals, material from a green vial was applied to one arm while another substance from a red vial was applied to the other arm. Unknown to the subjects, the green vial contained tuberculin, which is a harmless protein derived from the bacillus that causes tuberculosis, while the red vial contained saline. Tuberculin does not itself cause the disease, but in those who have been exposed to the bacillus beforehand, it triggers an inflammatory reaction. After six months, the contents of the vials were secretly reversed. This time, the arm to which the tuberculin was applied did not produce nearly such a vigorous inflammatory response. The volunteers had been conditioned to expect no inflammation to result from the material in the red vial, and their response to tuberculin was accordingly suppressed when it came out of the red container. The conditioning did not, however, work the other way round: the arm painted with the saline did not generate an inflammatory response, even when it came from the green vial.

It is still too early to say for sure, but studies like this suggest that immune conditioning evolved as a protective mechanism, to save the immune system from unnecessary expenditure, and not as a general-purpose learning mechanism to enable the immune system to respond in any way to any psychological input.

THE ORIGINS OF IMMUNITY

To claim that immune conditioning evolved as a protective mechanism is to assume that it evolved by natural selection. This is by no means the only possible evolutionary explanation for immune conditioning, however. It might simply have evolved by chance. As far as evolution is concerned, chance comes in several guises. One form of chance is known as 'random genetic drift'. A mutation arises that conveys no advantage to its bearers, but it spreads through the population anyway, by

sheer luck. Another form of chance is developmental entrenchment. The reason we have two kidneys and only one heart is
simply that, right from the very beginning, all vertebrates have
had two kidneys and one heart. This basic body plan has
acquired a kind of inertia; it is so deeply ingrained in the genes
that regulate embryonic development in all vertebrates that it
would be hard for evolution to change it.

It is unlikely that immune conditioning arose by random
genetic drift. Immune conditioning relies on a very complex set
of mechanisms that allow communication between the immune
system and the brain, and it is highly improbable that such
complex mechanisms would ever evolve simply by random
changes in gene frequency. However, the same consideration
does not rule out the possibility that immune conditioning
evolved by the other kind of chance. Complex mechanisms
that evolve by natural selection in a distant ancestor can be
retained by developmental entrenchment if they serve as vital
building blocks in embryonic development. Immune conditioning might be a mere side-effect of the fact that the very first
brains evolved in close contact with the immune system.

The immune system is far more ancient than the brain. It was,
in fact, one of the very first 'systems' to evolve. An organism can
only be analysed into different systems when it is composed of
more than one cell, and immune systems are found in the most
primitive of multicellular creatures. Sponges, for example, have
phagocytes (specialised cells designed for digesting foreign
material) which recognise bacteria and participate in wound
healing. These primitive immune cells defend sponges against
infection and tissue injury without any help or interference from
neurons, which sponges do not possess.

By the time neurons began to evolve, therefore, an immune
system of sorts was already well established. Indeed, the immune
system provided an important part of the physiological context
in which the first neurons appeared. In the first molluscs, for
example, which appeared around 550 million years ago, the
neurons did not form a discrete brain, but were rather clumped

in a number of clusters throughout the mollusc's sinewy body. There was therefore nothing to stop these neurons communicating freely with the immune cells, and indeed, this is what biologists observe in molluscs today. For example, when a mollusc comes into contact with a predator, the withdrawal reflex is triggered by the same signalling molecules that cause inflammation in mammals. First, the predator is detected by immune cells on the surface of the mollusc, which release IL-1. The IL-1 then binds to receptors on the mollusc's motor neurons, which initiate movement away from the threat. The immune system in molluscs thus functions as a kind of sensory organ.

Some biologists have suggested that the immune system also functions as a sensory organ in higher animals, including humans.[10] Just as the eyes allow us to detect light waves, so the immune system, like a sixth sense, enables us to detect the presence of the tiny invaders that constantly assail us from both within and without. In fact, it would be more accurate to call the immune system the 'first sense', since it is much older than vision and hearing, and should perhaps be classed as a form of touch.

With the appearance of the first vertebrates, the neurons linked up to form a single continuous web – the nervous system. The peripheral parts of this system fed information to its central part – the brain – which analysed the information and passed the new message back to the periphery. But the neurons retained their old affiliations with the cells of the immune system. They continued to speak in the same language, passing the same ancient signalling molecules back and forth. The fact that these molecules are classified by humans into neurotransmitters and immunotransmitters is largely a historical accident, depending on the system in which they were first detected. If a signalling molecule was first discovered in the brain, for example, it was designated a neurotransmitter. In reality, the same molecules that allow neurons to talk to each other also facilitate talk between neurons and immune cells. The same goes for the molecules that allow immune cells to communicate with each other.

With the evolution of the higher vertebrates, however, the conversation between the brain and the immune system became more difficult. The walls of blood vessels supplying the brain evolved special mechanisms to prevent the flow of all except the very smallest molecules from the blood to the brain. The blood–brain barrier, as it is called, protected the increasingly complex and vulnerable brain from all sorts of toxins and pathogens that might find their way into the bloodstream, but it also inhibited communication between the central nervous system and the immune cells in the periphery, since most of the signalling molecules that facilitate this communication process are too large to cross it. The fact that complex ways of bypassing this barrier then evolved – such as the chemical cascade described in Chapter Three, which allows a build up of IL-1 in the bloodstream to trigger an increase of IL-1 in the brain indirectly – suggests that the communication process was too important to allow the blood–brain barrier to get in the way. By this stage, a stunning variety of immune responses had evolved that could not function harmoniously without cerebral supervision. The immune system was simply no longer capable of the autonomy it once enjoyed, long ago, when it first evolved.

By the time of the appearance of the higher vertebrates in whom immune conditioning has been demonstrated, such as rats and dogs, the communication channels between the immune system and the brain were already well established. There never was, for example, an ancestral rat population in whom the immune system and the brain could not talk to each other. It is, therefore, perfectly possible that immune conditioning is simply a by-product of the immune–brain connections etched so deeply into the fundamental vertebrate body plan. Immune conditioning, in other words, might not have evolved to serve any function at all, whether protective or otherwise. The contingency of pure historical legacy, rather than natural selection, might be sufficient to explain why the immune systems of so many vertebrates can learn to suppress themselves in response to psychological stimuli.

This does not mean, of course, that immune conditioning could never be beneficial. It simply means that, whatever benefits immune conditioning may confer, these were not the reason it evolved. If immune conditioning is really just a by-product of the ancient connections between immune cells and neurons – connections that predate any kind of conditioning at all – then any benefits it may confer are merely fortuitous.

It could also be the case that immune conditioning is actually *dis*advantageous. If it really is just a by-product of neuro-immunological connections that are developmentally very entrenched in the vertebrate lineage, it might have survived despite consistently reducing chances of survival. Wherever possible, natural selection eliminates such disadvantageous traits, but sometimes there is simply no scope for natural selection to act because the disadvantageous trait is so deeply etched into the body plan. Perhaps the capacity for immune conditioning is like this.

THE PREHISTORY OF MEDICINE

Whatever the reason for the evolution of immune conditioning – whether it evolved by natural selection or by chance – it seems to be widespread among the higher vertebrates. By the time the human lineage began to diverge from that of the chimpanzees, some five million years ago, the capacity for immune conditioning was well established. Perhaps it was often triggered, or perhaps it was a latent capacity, lying dormant and rarely activated in reality. At some point, however, our ancestors discovered that they could activate it deliberately. They did not know exactly what they were doing, of course, but that is immaterial. The important thing is that they found, quite by chance, that they could train their immune systems to respond to certain stimuli in ways that felt quite beneficial. These stimuli – dabbing leaves on each other's wounds, perhaps, or giving each other special herbs when sick – were the origins of medicine.

When exactly this momentous event occurred, we do not really know. It must have been after the human lineage had already diverged from that of the chimpanzees, since chimpanzees do not practise medicine, if by medicine we mean the provision of special care to a sick individual *by others*. Primatologists have observed many cases in which a chimpanzee takes care of *himself* when ill or injured, sometimes in quite elaborate ways, such as consuming plants with medicinal properties or dabbing leaves on bloody wounds, but they have never seen one chimp providing this sort of medical assistance to another. Chimpanzees do spend long hours picking the ticks off each other's backs, which could, perhaps, be regarded as a kind of preventative medicine, but *therapeutic* medicine seems to lie outside their behavioural repertoire.

Archaeological evidence of ancient medical practices does not appear until relatively late. Ancient texts from Mesopotamia and Egypt provide written evidence that sophisticated medical practices were well established by 1700 BC,[11] but evidence of the existence of medicine prior to the advent of writing is much harder to come by. One rare example is the existence of skulls with small holes surrounded by calluses that indicate that trephining was being performed in places as far apart as France and the Pacific by 5000 BC. This is an operation involving cutting a small hole in the skull and scraping away portions of the cranium.[12] If such a complex operation was being performed seven thousand years ago, it is a fair bet that more primitive forms of medicine were being practised even earlier, but how much earlier is hard to say.

We know, then, that medicine – the provision of special care to the sick by others – must have originated some time between five million and ten thousand years ago. That is a very large time window. It is so large, in fact, as to leave us ignorant on the vital question of whether or not there has been enough time for natural selection to shape specific adaptations for medical care. If medicine originated towards the beginning of this window, shortly after the hominid lineage branched off from that of the chimpanzees, there would certainly have been time for the human brain to have developed special-purpose mechanisms for providing and responding to medical help. If, however, medicine only started towards the end of this time window, when our ancestors were already fully human, there would not have been time for any such special-purpose 'medical modules' to have evolved.

PAIN AS A NEED STATE

Even if we are ignorant on this point, we can still explore each of the alternatives. The first possibility is that medicine is a few million years old, and that humans have evolved special psychological mechanisms that are activated by the provision of medical attention. An intriguing suggestion as to what these mechanisms might comprise was put forward by the British physiologist Patrick Wall in the 1990s. Wall argued that the mechanisms underlying pain have evolved to be much more complex in humans than in other animals. Whereas in other, less complex animals the level of pain is determined simply by the amount of bodily damage, in humans it is also influenced by a whole range of factors in the social environment. Among these factors, Wall claimed, is the availability of medical help.

This, at least, seems to be what Wall meant when he claimed that pain is a 'need state', like hunger and thirst.[13] Need states are terminated by a specific consummatory act: hunger by eating, thirst by drinking. Pain, too, can be terminated by various 'consummatory acts'. Withdrawing one's hand rapidly from a hot stove is one such act; keeping a sprained ankle still is another. Crucial to Wall's argument, however, is that pain can sometimes be terminated simply by care and attention from others. It is this addition of a purely social event to the list of various consummatory acts relevant to pain that makes human pain such an evolutionary novelty.

Wall's claim about the relevance of social support to pain

relief is supported by the studies we looked at in Chapter Two that investigated the anti-inflammatory effects of fake ultrasound. One of these studies found that the placebo response was only triggered when the fake ultrasound was applied by *someone else*. When exactly the same physical stimulus was applied by the patients to their own faces, the swelling was not reduced. This suggests that the mere provision of social support can be sufficient to trigger the placebo response. Perhaps this is the result of natural selection wiring up the pain-generating circuits in the brain to inputs from the neural regions that are sensitive to social support. This, of course, presupposes that medical care has been a feature of our environment for long enough to enable such evolutionary change to take place.

If Wall's theory is right, and natural selection has designed specific brain circuits to feed information about the social environment into the circuits that generate pain, such circuits must confer some evolutionary advantage on those who have them. It is hard, however, to see what this advantage might be. As we have already seen, pain is a vital protective mechanism, and those who lack the capacity to feel pain do not survive very long. What possible advantage could there be in having a mechanism that shuts down pain when medical care – and perhaps other kinds of social assistance too – is provided? Surely it would be better to make the sensation of pain autonomous, independent of such social factors?

Not necessarily. There are costs as well as benefits associated with pain. In particular, high levels of pain can actually slow down the healing process. When one is alone, the protective value of pain might outweigh the disadvantage of slowing down the healing process, but when others are taking care of you, the cost–benefit ratio may change. In particular, when others can protect you, pain might not be so vital. In effect, medical care might allow the patient to offload the protective function of pain onto others: self-defence is unnecessary when other people are around to do the defending for you. If this is true, then a person whose brain was capable of shutting down pain when it detected the presence of medical help might actually have an advantage over someone whose brain lacked this capacity.

EXTENDING THE IDEA

Wall's theory applies just to pain, and so, while it might help to explain the evolution of placebo analgesia, it cannot explain why the placebo response should affect other phenomena. Nevertheless, it might be possible to extend Wall's theory to other aspects of the placebo response. Perhaps the neural mechanisms that detect the provision of medical care do not simply feed into a circuit dedicated to pain (which, incidentally, is not neurologically plausible) but to a more general neural mechanism dedicated to the whole range of phenomena associated with the acute phase response. When medical care arrives on the scene, such mechanisms would be able to suppress not just pain, but all the other aspects of the acute phase response too – from swelling and fever to lethargy and loss of appetite.

The mechanisms that suppress the acute phase response are as little understood as those involved in the placebo response. It is known, however, that the body possesses a number of potent chemicals that inhibit the generation and operation of the key cytokines involved. The precise role of endorphins in this process is not well understood, but they too may help damp down the acute phase response. In the normal run of events, the acute phase response generally subsides between three and four days after infection or injury, but if the mechanisms responsible for suppressing it can be activated by the arrival of social care, then the placebo effect may simply be a way to bring forward the normal process of termination. In fact, this may even be the evolutionary origin of the placebo response. In Chapter Three, we saw how the innate immune system and the acquired immune system are, to some extent, antagonistic. When bacteria have entered the body, the macrophages that are part of the innate immune system start to attack them by secreting nitric oxide, which slows down the rate at which bacteria divide. However, the nitric oxide also slows down the division of T-cells and B-cells, which form the backbone of the acquired immune response. The extra delay caused to the acquired immune response by the secretion of nitric oxide is not in itself adaptive, but it is a price worth paying to keep the bacteria at bay in the early stages of infection. The dangers of allowing the bacteria to get too much of a head start before the acquired immune system can mount its counter-attack must be great, especially if the energy and resources required by the acquired immune system are in short supply.

If there were situations in which it was a good idea to suppress the acute phase earlier than normal, thus allowing the acquired immune system to kick in more rapidly, then any organism that could detect them and suppress the acute phase accordingly would have an advantage.

IMMUNE TRAFFICKING

This hypothesis assumes that the placebo response is a specific adaptation that natural selection has designed to allow humans to respond appropriately to the provision of medical care. However, this is to presuppose that medicine has been around long enough for natural selection to alter our neural design accordingly. And, as we have already seen, this is by no means certain. Medicine might well be that ancient; but it could also be under ten thousand years old, which is too short a time for natural selection to have crafted special neural circuitry for responding to medical help. If medicine turns out to be this recent, then Wall's theory of pain as a need state designed to motivate the search for medical help, and the adaptive story of the placebo response we just constructed on the basis of this theory, cannot be true. If medicine is an evolutionary novelty, the placebo response cannot have evolved by natural selection. It would, rather, have to be a mere by-product of something that evolved for another reason.

If the placebo response is simply a by-product, then it is probably a by-product of immune conditioning. This does not mean that the placebo response is just another name for immune conditioning, however. As already noted, some researchers have assumed this position, but there are several reasons why it is not a very helpful view. Chief among these is the fact that immune conditioning is a much broader category than the placebo response. All sorts of immune activity can be conditioned, including activation of the inflammatory response. The placebo effect, however, seems to be restricted to suppression of the inflammatory response, and so is probably best seen as just one particular kind of immune conditioning.

Earlier in this chapter, we asked whether immune conditioning itself evolved by natural selection, or whether it too is a by-product of some yet more ancient structure. We also speculated that, if immune conditioning did evolve by natural selection, its function might be to protect the immune system from harmful immunosuppressive toxins. The idea is that white blood cells and other immune agents might be such precious resources that it would be wasteful to allow them to circulate around the body when they would be destroyed by toxins. Any animal, then, that could respond to the presence of toxins in the bloodstream by withdrawing its immune resources from peripheral circulation and locking them away safely in organs such as the thymus, would have an advantage over animals that could not.

There is, in fact, growing evidence that such 'trafficking' of white blood cells between the peripheral circulation and the central organs of the immune system, does occur. The immune system, it appears, can regulate the proportion of various kinds of white blood cells that circulate freely around the body and the proportion of those that are locked up in the thymus and the lymph nodes. Depending on the circumstances, more white blood cells can be released into the peripheral circulation, or quickly shunted back again into their 'home' organs. Perhaps this is all that is going on in the case of immune conditioning. We know that conditioning can lead to suppression of the immune system because we can measure the number of various kinds of white cells in the bloodstream, and this number drops sharply in response to various conditioned stimuli. We should ask, however, what happens to the white blood cells that have disappeared. They cannot simply have died; the fall in number is too rapid for that. Rather, these cells must have gone somewhere else in the body. It seems highly likely that conditioned immunosuppression simply involves moving certain immune agents out of the bloodstream and into the safety of various organs.

HUMPHREY'S REMEDY

The British psychologist Nicholas Humphrey has proposed an evolutionary theory of the placebo response that expands on the idea that it involves the safeguarding of precious immune resources.[14] Whenever we observe a placebo response, he argues, we can infer that a latent capacity for self-cure was being actively *inhibited* beforehand. Humphrey recognises that this hypothesis implies some counterintuitive theses. For example, it implies that when self-cure is inhibited, there must be good reason for this under the existing circumstances. In other words, there must be circumstances under which it is better to remain sick than to heal oneself, either because there are benefits to remaining sick, or because there are costs to the process of self-cure.

As an example of the costs of self-healing, Humphrey cites evidence showing that the immune system is a very expensive piece of machinery to maintain. For example, the production of antibodies uses up a surprisingly large amount of metabolic energy, and requires a continual supply of quite rare nutrients in the diet, such as carotenoids. And, as with any powerful drug, immune agents can have nasty side-effects, such as auto-immune diseases. The moral is clear: immune agents should be used with great care. One thing the body should *not* do, when it first detects an infectious agent, is to throw everything it has at the invader.

Humphrey's model explains the placebo response in the following way. When someone is sick, they use their internal healing resources sparingly, for the reasons already outlined: these resources are expensive, and cannot be replenished very easily, so should not be squandered. It is always wise to keep some in reserve. The arrival of medical attention, however, changes the picture somewhat. Medical treatment provides a fairly reliable signal to the patient that recovery is around the corner. There is a good chance that the patient is not in for a protracted battle against the disease, and will soon have a chance to replenish the waning stock of internal healing resources. In view of this, it is no longer so important to keep a large amount of these resources in reserve. The patient can now throw everything he's got at the injury or disease. And this is what lies behind the placebo response.

Humphrey's theory differs from the one advanced in this book in a few details. For one thing, the prototypical placebo response envisioned in Humphrey's account is one in which a sick person liberates a wealth of precious immune agents – antibodies and so on – that had previously been sequestered away in some safe house in the body such as the thymus. Yet, as should be clear by now, most, if not all, genuine cases of the placebo response involve precisely the opposite – the suppression of an immune response, rather than its activation. And the kind of immune response that is suppressed does not tend to involve antibodies and other aspects of the acquired immune system, but rather the elements of the innate immune system. To be fair to Humphrey, it should be pointed out that his theory was developed at a higher level of abstraction that was not committed to any particular hypothesis about the biological mechanisms involved.

Another difference is that Humphrey thinks the placebo response is triggered not so much by a belief as by *hope*. If a belief is involved, it is a very general kind of belief, to the effect that recovery is just around the corner, or that good times are on their way, or some other grounds for optimism. There is no reason why, in Humphrey's account, we should expect placebo responses to be limited to the context of medical assistance. Anything that provides grounds for hope – whether it be medical care or winning the lottery – should be capable, at least in principle, of encouraging the immune system to be more liberal with its precious resources. This is rather different from the view proposed in the previous chapter, according to which the crucial trigger for the placebo response is the belief that one has received powerful medicine.

More important than these points of divergence, however, are the similarities between Humphrey's views and my own. Both theories emphasise the importance of viewing the placebo response in the context of a more general problem – that of how the organism manages its own immune resources. The metaphor of management is apt. Humphrey even talks of a 'natural healthcare management system', and compares it to managed healthcare. But then the convergence is hardly an accident, as Humphrey's suggestive paper on 'The Evolutionary Psychology of Faith Healing and the Placebo Effect' was one of the original sources of inspiration for this book.

Chapter 6

NOCEBO — BEYOND GOOD AND BAD

The ultimate dream of pharmacology must surely be the drug that has no side-effects. Such an idea will always remain a fantasy, of course, since the complexity of biological systems virtually guarantees that any attempt to tinker with one element will have unintended consequences elsewhere. For all the contemporary rhetoric about 'rational drug design' and 'magic bullets', the various medicines we ingest and inject remain incredibly blunt instruments. Part of the problem lies in getting the active ingredient to the place where it is needed. Most drugs are taken orally, which means that they must first pass through the digestive tract, and then the liver, where they will be absorbed into the bloodstream, and affect millions of other cells all over the body before finally — one hopes — reaching the intended target. Drugs that are injected directly into the bloodstream or the cerebrospinal fluid may circumvent the digestive tract, but they still affect a lot of other areas besides the one for which they are meant. At the moment, and for the foreseeable future, there is no easy way to ensure that, say, an antidepressant goes straight to the brain and nowhere else.

Even if this problem is solved, and scientists discover better ways of delivering active ingredients to the precise area of the body where they are needed, and nowhere else, it is unlikely that side-effects will be eliminated. Once a drug has reached the area of the body for which it is intended, it must still get inside the cells and interfere with the complex network of chemical reactions going on there. The precise nature of this network depends on the type of cell, what point of the life-cycle the cell happens to be at, and the nature of the cell's local environment. Biologists have traced some of these networks, and their schematic diagrams resemble intricate spiders' webs of baffling interconnections, like the wiring diagrams for a machine designed by a mad scientist. And this is just the tip of the iceberg: compared to the vastness of what remains to be discovered, our current knowledge of cellular functioning is a tiny beachhead in a dark and mysterious continent.

Of one thing, however, we can be certain. Any attempt to interfere with one element in the network of intracellular reactions will have numerous and unpredictable consequences downstream. The claims put out by various pharmaceutical companies to have discovered 'smart drugs' resemble the news-peak of certain military authorities whose 'smart bombs' result in embarrassingly large amounts of 'collateral damage'. In fact, one might propose the principle that the more effective a drug is, the more likely it is to have powerful and potentially harmful side-effects, as the first law of pharmacology.

THE SIDE-EFFECTS OF PLACEBOS

For some writers, placebos are a shining exception to the first law of pharmacology. According to Robert Buckman and Karl Sabbagh, for example, placebos 'have some effect on almost every symptom known to man', but 'have no side-effects and cannot be given in overdose'.[1] Yet, elsewhere in the same book, Buckman and Sabbagh also claim (in what amounts to a restatement of the first law of pharmacology) that a non-toxic drug is bound to be ineffective.[2] Surely they cannot have it both ways. If the first law is correct, then either placebos are powerful – in which case they can also be dangerous – or placebos have no side-effects – in which case they are useless.

The whole question of side-effects is yet another of the many areas of confusion that have dogged research into the placebo effect from its earliest days. As one might expect, Beecher himself got the topic off to a bad start. Realising, perhaps, that it would be rather implausible to argue that placebos could do much good but no harm, he stated that 'not only do placebos produce beneficial effects, but like other therapeutic agents they have associated toxic effects'.[3] But the evidence on which he based this statement was as flawed as that on which he based his claims for the therapeutic powers of placebos. In both cases, he simply assumed that anything experienced by subjects in the placebo arm of a clinical trial was the direct effect of the placebo. If people in the placebo group got better, Beecher assumed that this was because the placebo had helped them. If they reported a dry mouth, or a headache, this was interpreted as a 'side-effect'. In both cases, the assumption was unjustified. Just as there will be a certain proportion of patients in any group who get better without any help, there will also be a certain number who get dry mouths and headaches anyway, even in the absence of any powerful drugs.

To provide good evidence for placebogenic side-effects, of course, we would have to compare the experience of those in a placebo group with that of people in a no-treatment group. Only if those given a placebo had significantly more headaches, for example, than those not given a placebo, could we be sure that placebos are capable of causing headaches – and so on for every one of the other so-called 'side-effects' that Beecher attributed to placebos. Without such a no-treatment control group, the figures Beecher quoted in his paper – 9 per cent felt nauseous after taking a placebo, 25 per cent got headaches, and so on – mean nothing. All but one of these studies involved people who were sick, and such people would be expected to show such symptoms anyway.

Despite these clear flaws, Beecher's remarks about the capacity of placebos to induce side-effects went unchallenged. By the 1970s the idea was so well-entrenched among medical researchers that it was regarded as a fact that should be 'demonstrated' to medical students, rather than as a hypothesis to be tested. In 1972, for example, teachers at one medical school in the United States set up a class experiment in which students were asked to volunteer for a study to investigate 'the psychological and physiological effects of stimulant and sedative drugs'.[4] Volunteers were randomly allocated to four treatment groups, in which each person was given either one or two pink or blue capsules. Unknown to the volunteers, the capsules contained no active substance. Volunteers completed a self-assessment form to evaluate their psychological state, and carried out a few basic physiological observations on each other, both immediately before taking the capsules and then one hour afterwards. Between taking the capsules and carrying out the second set of observations, the volunteers attended a one-hour lecture.

Sure enough, when the two sets of measurements were compared, it was found that many of the students had undergone changes in their psychological and physiological states. After presenting these results to the students, the teachers then announced, dramatically, that the capsules had in fact been placebos. The students were duly impressed, and rated the experience highly for its learning value. 'The object of our study,' reported the teachers in their subsequent paper, 'was to convince medical students of the placebo effect,' and this, it seems, they achieved. Yet this achievement depended on hiding from the students some serious flaws in the experimental set-up – the very same flaws that marred Beecher's own hasty conclusions about the side-effects of placebos. Once again, no control group was used. The students who did not volunteer to take the capsules were not given the psychological and physiological tests before and after the lecture, so we cannot be sure that those taking the placebos underwent any greater changes than those who did not. Indeed, the most common changes experienced by those who took the capsules – drowsiness, sluggishness and tiredness – were just those that anyone might report after sitting through an hour-long lecture!

More recent studies have tended to repeat these methodological errors. In 1993, for example, a meta-analysis investigated the topic of side-effects by pooling the results of 109 placebo-controlled studies.[5] Like the 'demonstration to medical students' (and unlike Beecher's original paper), this meta-analysis focused entirely on trials involving healthy volunteers who would be less likely to have symptoms anyway. However, even healthy people experience headaches and other mild symptoms from time to time, so a no-placebo control group would still be needed to justify claims that such symptoms were the direct result of being given placebos. Yet no comparative data was included in the meta-analysis. Rather, the authors simply assumed that any 'adverse events' reported by the people taking placebos must be due to the placebo itself, just as Beecher had done.

Despite the flaw in its central assumption, the 1993 meta-analysis did contain some slightly more persuasive data. The authors also compared the number of symptoms reported by subjects receiving a single dose of placebo with the number of adverse events reported by those receiving multiple doses. While this is certainly not as good as comparing a placebo group with a no-treatment group, it does at least provide some comparative data. If the placebo response is dose-dependent, then more side-effects should presumably be reported by those taking multiple doses. There were, indeed, some small differences of this kind. Those receiving repeated doses of placebo were slightly more likely to report headaches, weakness, dizziness and nausea (and, strangely, less likely to report drowsiness).

There are various reasons why these results should be treated with a certain degree of caution. For one thing, the single-dose and multiple-dose placebo groups were taken from different studies, so we cannot be sure that the people in each group were really comparable. Nevertheless, the fact that the subjects in all the studies were healthy volunteers probably rules out most of the possible differences. As scientists never tire of saying, 'more research is needed'. Still, it does seem that there are some grounds for thinking that placebos can induce mild symptoms such as headaches, nausea and weakness.

WHEN BELIEF KILLS

If it is true that placebos really are capable of inducing such symptoms, this would seem to pose a problem for the claim, advanced in Chapter Three, that placebos work by suppressing the acute phase response. For headaches, nausea and feelings of weakness are typically associated with the activation of the acute phase response, not its suppression. Indeed, it was the fact that placebos generally tend to *relieve* such symptoms that led us to explore the possibility that placebos suppress the acute phase response in the first place. Now, it seems, placebos can also *produce* such symptoms. Does this mean that placebos are not exclusively suppressive? Can the placebo response also involve the *activation* of the innate immune system?

This is in part a semantic issue. If we simply *define* the placebo response as the suppression of the acute phase response, the hypothesis is saved, for then the headaches would simply not count as part of the placebo response. This would be a hollow victory. What we are really interested in is how beliefs can affect the immune system, not in the words we use to describe these influences. Nevertheless, there is some value in making the right distinctions, even if only to facilitate communication and avoid misunderstanding. Some medical researchers, indeed, use a different term − the *nocebo effect* − to refer to the process whereby adverse events like headaches are produced by inert medication.

Although this phrase is clearly reminiscent of the word *placebo*, and has a similarly classical etymology (*nocebo* is Latin for 'I shall harm'), it is in fact much more recent, appearing in the medical literature for the first time in the 1960s.[6] Yet this terminological innovation did not clarify the confused thinking about placebos; in fact, it made things even worse. For one thing, it perpetuated the misleading impression that the good, or bad, effects observed in those given, say, a sugar pill, are due to the pill itself, rather than to the beliefs of the person taking it. Just as the placebo response is caused by the belief that some effective help has been given, rather than by the placebo itself, so the nocebo effect is caused by the belief that some harmful process has been administered, rather than by the nocebo itself. Here again, it might be more helpful to talk about the 'belief effect', rather than the placebo or nocebo effect.

Some evidence for the key role of belief in the nocebo effect is provided by the mysterious phenomenon known as 'voodoo death'. This term was coined by the distinguished British physiologist Walter Cannon in 1942, but the phenomenon itself has been known about for centuries.[7] In diverse cultures, from Africa and South America to Asia and Australia, many competent authorities have reported cases in which people have died within a few days of a voodoo priest or witch doctor pronouncing a ritual curse upon them. Crucial to the efficacy of such curses is the knowledge that it has been cast, and the belief that it works. Curses do not work if the victim is unaware of them, and they are equally useless if the victim is not superstitious. Voodoo death would seem, then, to be a clear case of the belief effect.

Perhaps we should not be quite so quick to come to this conclusion. We can only speak of the belief effect when a belief has a direct impact on the immune system. As noted earlier, beliefs can affect one's health via a number of other less direct routes too. The most obvious example of such an indirect route is behaviour. If a superstitious person believes that a curse has been placed upon him, he might lose the will to live, stop eating, and die of self-neglect. This would not be a case of the belief effect because the superstitious belief would not have affected the immune system directly, but indirectly, via its effect on the person's behaviour.

Unfortunately, there is not enough evidence to decide whether the various reported cases of voodoo death are really examples of the belief effect, or whether they involve something much simpler, such as changes in behaviour. But this difficulty does illustrate the need for much clearer thinking about the whole issue of psychosomatic disease. Many sick people have negative thoughts, but we cannot conclude from this fact alone that their illnesses are *caused* by some kind of direct psychological interference with their immune systems. Perhaps their pessimism has simply led them to take less care of themselves. It is also quite likely – perhaps even more so – that the causal arrow runs in the other direction: the illness may induce the negative thoughts, rather than the other way round.

THE AMBIGUITY OF HEALTH AND DISEASE

In coining a new term – the nocebo effect – to describe the way that dummy treatments could trigger symptoms as well as relieving them, medical researchers not only obscured the role of beliefs in this process, but also helped to strengthen the simplistic dichotomy between the 'good' and 'bad' effects of medical treatment. In doing so, they failed to grasp one of the most important lessons that research into placebos has to teach us – that our current understanding of what constitutes good and bad health is terribly confused.

For most people, good health is equivalent to 'feeling good', and bad health is equivalent to 'feeling bad'. According to this view, it would be quite coherent to divide the effects of dummy treatments into 'placebo effects' and 'nocebo effects', depending on whether they make you feel better or worse. If a sugar pill takes away your pain, or reduces swelling, it must be a placebo. If, on the other hand, it gives you a headache or makes you feel nauseous, it must be a nocebo. It all sounds very straightforward. It should be clear by now, though, that this way of thinking is far too simplistic.

Take pain, for example. Pain is often a sign that something is wrong with the body. But this does not mean that pain itself is part of the problem. Quite the opposite. As we saw in Chapter Three, pain is a valuable protective mechanism. The brain generates short, sharp bursts of pain to make us withdraw rapidly from damaging objects, and creates long-lasting, dull pain to make us refrain from moving wounded areas. Without the pain, our lives would be less unpleasant, but it is likely that they would also be considerably shorter.

Pain, then, is actually a healthy thing — and this is true not because of any Calvinistic belief in the value of suffering *per se*. The injury it signals is not healthy, but the signal itself is. This is why blocking pain with morphine — or, indeed, a placebo — can be a very risky business. By removing this protective signal, painkillers of any kind can prevent people from guarding injured areas, which can delay healing or even postpone it indefinitely. The same principle probably applies to all the other aspects of the acute phase response. Blocking fever with antipyretic drugs, for example, has been shown to reduce the capacity to fight infection. It is likely that abolishing the feelings of lethargy and apathy that often accompany illness by giving stimulants to sick people would also have detrimental effects, but this idea has not yet been tested experimentally.

These facts have far reaching implications. They challenge us to reconsider the whole way we think about health and disease. When feeling bad is seen in the context of the body's adaptive response to injury and infection, medical treatments that simply abolish those feelings can no longer be seen as unambiguously beneficial. Likewise, the unpleasant symptoms triggered by some treatments might not always be undesirable 'side-effects', but may be part and parcel of their therapeutic action. In the wider context of the organism's ability to cope with biological and psychological dangers, the costs and benefits of feeling bad are often rather different to how we might first imagine them.

These considerations apply just as much to dummy treatments as to real ones. If the placebo response works by suppressing the acute phase response before it would naturally subside, then perhaps placebos too are not as harmless as some researchers have thought. Certainly, it does not seem very useful to classify the effects of dummy treatments into placebo effects and nocebo effects simply on the basis of whether or not they make us feel better or worse. Rather, the effects of dummy treatments need to be understood in terms of the underlying biological mechanisms that they trigger, and of the role these mechanisms play in fighting infection and protecting us from injury.

THE TOXIC THEORY OF MEDICINE

If dummy treatments can activate various elements of the acute phase response as well as suppressing them, why is it that – most of the time – they seem to do the former rather than the latter? Why is it, in other words, that placebos have generally been associated with relieving pain rather than increasing it, and on the rare occasions when the opposite has been observed, people have felt the need to designate this phenomenon with a separate term? One possibility, which was mooted in the previous chapter, is that this linguistic practice is in accord with some deeper evolutionary logic. That would be the case if the placebo response evolved just to suppress the acute phase response, and the rare occasions when the reverse occurs is just some fortuitous by-product. This, however, presupposes that the practice of giving medical care has been around for long enough for natural selection to shape a specific biological adaptation for responding to it. And this, as we have seen, is by no means certain.

If medical care is a relatively recent phenomenon, emerging less than ten thousand years ago, then we must seek an alternative explanation for why placebos generally suppress immune responses rather than activating them. We are once again deep into the realm of speculation, but it is nonetheless interesting to explore the various possibilities. One possible explanation, in particular, deserves some attention, as it bears directly on the paradoxical relationship between feeling good and being healthy that we have been looking at in this chapter. We might call it the toxic theory of medicine.

Very briefly, the idea is as follows. Most medical treatments, from the very earliest times through to the golden age of scientific medicine in the latter part of the twentieth century, have worked by blocking the body's natural defence mechanisms rather than enhancing them. Painkillers are the most obvious example. Over 95 per cent of the painkillers used by doctors today are based on derivatives from just two natural herbal remedies that have been in use for hundreds of years: opium and aspirin.[8] Opium, in fact, has been used in Asia for over three millennia, though not always for purely medical reasons. Aspirin is derived from the bark of the white willow tree, which the Reverend Edmund Stone of Chipping Norton reported to have powerful anti-inflammatory and antipyretic effects in 1763. (Stone was apparently unaware that Hippocrates and Galen had also recommended the use of willow bark). Despite their key role in medicine, both these drugs are now known to work by suppressing various aspects of immune activity.

The opiates, which include morphine and heroin, work — as we have already seen — by blocking the very receptors that evolved to allow our brains to modulate the pain signal carried by nerves from damaged tissue. They are also known to have other effects, which include damping down various aspects of the innate immune response. Aspirin also interferes with the acute phase response, as it blocks the action of a family of molecules — the prostaglandins — that play a key role in producing swelling, fever and blood clotting.

Cannabis, too, has been used for thousands of years to relieve pain. The Assyrians, Indians and Chinese all used it in various medical procedures, and it is also mentioned in an ancient Egyptian medical papyrus dating from 1550 BC. Traces of burned cannabis have been found in the chest cavity of a female skeleton discovered at Beith Shamesh in Israel, dated to the fourth century BC. The young woman almost certainly died in childbirth, as the skeleton of a full-term foetus was found trapped in her pelvic area, and the cannabis was probably used as a way of relieving the pain of labour.[9] Yet cannabis too is now known to suppress certain aspects of immune activity.

It is not just the ancient remedies that turn out to be immunosuppressive. Even the wonder drugs of the twentieth century have, by and large, been found to work by damping down various aspects of the body's natural defence systems. Cortisone, for example, which came into widespread use in the late 1940s and is now used in treating a vast array of conditions from rheumatoid and skin disorders to various forms of cancer and brain disease, is simply a kind of steroid, and – as we saw in Chapter Three – steroids are known to suppress the innate immune response, at least at the high dosage levels found in most medical treatments. Unlike aspirin, which affects only the prostaglandin element of the inflammatory response, steroids have a much broader effect, damping down a whole range of cytokines, including IL-1. This is why steroids can have such terrible side-effects. As one doctor commented, reflecting on the introduction of steroids in the late 1940s, 'my generation will never forget the severe complications they produced – the moon face, the perforated and bleeding ulcers, the bruising and crushed vertebrae.'[10]

In fact, the list of medical treatments that work reads like a litany of immunosuppressive agents. Chemotherapy attacks cancer tumours, but it also destroys immune cells. Surgery removes diseased tissue, but also often introduces new infections. Vaccination, which stimulates the immune system to produce antibodies, is the exception that proves the rule. And when we add to this list the vast number of discredited remedies from bygone ages that actually made things worse – bloodletting, leeching and so on – the toxic theory of medicine becomes even more persuasive. Consider, for example, the treatment of Charles II by his team of distinguished doctors, who, we may suppose, provided him with the best medical attention money could buy in the seventeenth century:

> The King was bled . . . to the extent of a pint from his right arm. Next [the physician] drew eight ounces of blood from the left shoulder . . . gave an emetic to make the King vomit, two physics, and an enema containing antimony, rock salt, marshmallow leaves, violets, beet root, camomile flowers, fennel seed, linseed, cardamom seed, cinnamon, saffron, cochineal, and aloes.

The King's head was then shaved and a blister raised on his scalp. A sneezing powder of hellebore root was given to purge his brain, and a powder of cowslip administered to strengthen it, for it was the belief in those days that the nasal secretion came from the brain. The emetics were continued at frequent intervals and meanwhile a soothing drink was given, composed of barley water, licorice, and sweet almonds, light wine, oil of wormwood, anise, thistle leaves, mint, rose, and angelica. A plaster of pitch and pigeon dung was put on the King's feet. Next there was more bleeding followed by the administration of melon seeds, manna, slippery elm, black cherry water, extract of lily of the valley, peony, lavender, pearls dissolved in vinegar, gentian root, nutmeg, and cloves. To this mixture were added forty drops of the extract of human skull. Finally in desperation a bezoar stone was tried. The King died.[11]

If medical care has, since its very inception, tended to be so invariably toxic, it is hardly surprising that people have learnt to respond to it by suppressing their immune responses. This might be the reason why placebos tend to damp down the immune system rather than boosting it. Far from being a specific adaptation designed by natural selection, the placebo response might simply be the result of a more general mechanism – that of immune conditioning – interacting with a long cultural tradition of bashing the acute phase response whenever it manifested itself.

FEVER PHOBIA

Doctors today are much more aware of the adaptive value of the body's natural response to illness. They are correspondingly less likely to blitz the patient with painkillers and other immunosuppressive drugs whenever he reports feeling ill. Professional medicine may, then, finally be emerging from its long association with toxic interventions. But it may take some time before this attitude spreads to the population as a whole. For if medical assistance has so long concentrated on suppressing elements of the body's natural defences, this has not been entirely the fault of doctors. The great majority of ordinary people have actively colluded in the toxic theory of medicine. Which person, in pain, has not automatically reached for the nearest available painkiller – whether it be a modern analgesic such as aspirin, or an ancient one such as opium?

Popular attitudes to fever are a case in point – particularly when the victim of the fever is a child. Fever is one of the most common reasons that parents seek medical attention for their children, a habit that is almost certainly due to the widespread belief that fever is a disease rather than the body's way of fighting infection. In 1980, the American physician Barton Schmitt coined the term 'fever phobia' to designate the numerous misconceptions parents had about fever.[12] Schmitt found that 63 per cent of caregivers were worried a great deal that serious harm could result from fevers, and 18 per cent believed that brain damage could be caused by mild fevers of only 38.9 degrees celsius or less – both views which were, even then, wildly exaggerated by the standards of proper medical evidence. Two decades later, a team of paediatricians from Johns Hopkins Bayview Medical Center in Baltimore found that attitudes had not changed much.[13] Concern about fever and its potential harmful effects repeatedly led parents to excessive monitoring and aggressive treatment, including sponging with cool water (which can cause significant shivering, as a result of the body attempting to stay warm) or even alcohol (which can cause dehydration and hypoglycaemia, particularly in young children). The team of researchers found that parents are even more dangerously liberal with fever-reducing drugs than they were two decades ago, giving high doses of acetaminophen and ibuprofen, placing their children at undue risk of toxicity. Interestingly, 29 per cent of the people surveyed said that they followed the recommendations of the American Academy of Paediatrics, despite the fact that no such policy exists! Clearly it would be unfair to lay all the blame for toxic medicine at the hands of medical professionals.

WHEN DOES PAIN STOP BEING A GOOD THING?

The toxic theory calls into doubt the grand claims advanced on behalf of medicine. The 'greatest benefit to mankind', as medicine has been called, might not be so unambiguously beneficial. However, it would be a mistake to swing to the opposite extreme, as some do, and conclude that medicine is entirely a Bad Thing. Jehovah's Witnesses are forbidden by their religion to accept certain kinds of medical care on the grounds that it interferes with God's will. Many New Age gurus and devotees of alternative medicine are also highly sceptical of orthodox medicine, though they do not usually go to the same extremes as the Jehovah's Witnesses in refusing vital blood transfusions. Their belief that orthodox medicine is somehow 'unnatural' is, however, not a million miles away from the religious scruples of the Witnesses.

The truth is that, however paradoxical it may sound, even toxic medicine can sometimes be good for you. If it were not, it would surely have fizzled out long ago. Suppressing the body's natural defence mechanisms is certainly a bad thing in many situations, but there are occasions when these mechanisms malfunction, and turn against the body they are supposed to protect. In these circumstances, blocking the defence mechanisms is the best thing you can do.

Pain, once again, provides the best example. In the normal run of events, pain is — as we have already seen — a valuable protective system. As with any other biological response, however, the systems that generate pain do occasionally go wrong. Sometimes, the brain generates pain that is completely useless. The pain caused by cancer, for example, is of no protective value at all, since the disease only causes pain when it is quite advanced. In such cases, there is absolutely nothing to be gained by allowing the pain to persist, and doctors can therefore administer painkillers to cancer patients without any scruples.

The problem is that, with the exception of such obvious examples as this, it is very hard to be sure that any particular pain is useless. The brain is often cleverer than we are, and it may be generating the pain for a good reason that we cannot figure out. The same applies to the other aspects of the acute phase response. Sometimes fever can reach levels that are not only dangerous to the invading bacteria, which is the purpose of the fever, but also to the sick person himself, which is most definitely a malfunction. Yet it is very hard to know exactly when the costs of the fever begin to outweigh the benefits. Once upon a time, doctors assumed that all fever was bad, and sought to abolish it in any way they could. Now they know slightly better, but they are still ignorant of many of the details. Exactly how high does someone's temperature have to be before it is better to give him an antipyretic drug rather than letting him sweat it out? The biological costs and benefits are often too complex to calculate exactly.

And, of course, there is the problem of side-effects again. Even when we are sure that a person's temperature has risen so high as to be more of a threat than a benefit, the antipyretic drugs we give him have many effects besides reducing fever. Aspirin, for example, interferes with blood clotting as well, and so can trigger fatal haemorrhages. Sometimes, on the other hand, excessive blood clotting is the problem, as when clots in the coronary arteries cause heart attacks, and in such cases the anti-clotting effects of aspirin are beneficial. Everything depends on the precise nature of the problem and the details of the mechanism that is malfunctioning.

THE BENEFITS OF STOMACH ULCERS

It should be clear by now that it can be much harder than is generally realised to distinguish between symptoms that indicate genuine pathology and those that are vital elements of the body's own defences. First impressions are often misleading. Pain and fever feel bad, but that does not mean we should always try to suppress them. The placebo effect and the nocebo effect refer to the same biological process – the suppression of the acute phase response. Sometimes, this can be a good thing, but at other times it may not.

The double-edged nature of symptoms like pain and fever is already well established, but there are intriguing suggestions that the same basic principle may hold for many other conditions that have, up to now at least, been regarded as unambiguously pernicious. Stomach ulcers are a case in point. Ever since the medical community decided, in the 1980s, that ulcers were caused by bacterial infection, tremendous efforts have been made in some countries to eliminate the bacterium responsible, *Helicobacter pylori*. Patients with stomach ulcers in many Western countries are now routinely treated with antibiotics, and as a result *H. pylori* infection rates have plummeted. The race is now on for a vaccine that will wipe out *H. pylori* once and for all. Since *H. pylori* is also thought to cause a kind of stomach cancer known as gastric carcinoma, scientists hope that such a vaccine would not only prevent ulcers, but also reduce levels of cancer.

Towards the end of the 1990s, however, some researchers began to uncover evidence that suggested *H. pylori* might not be the pure villain it has been made out to be. In 1999, for example, Swedish researchers discovered that *H. pylori* produces substances that kill other bacteria such as *E. coli*.[14] The following year, a team of scientists in Germany found evidence that those infected with *H. pylori* had lower rates of diarrhoea than those who were not. There are even reports that the bacterium may protect against a kind of stomach cancer known as oesophageal adenocarcinoma. This type of cancer is usually quite rare, but it has been rapidly increasing in frequency in just those countries where *H. pylori* infection has fallen due to the use of antibiotics.[15]

If *H. pylori* can protect us against bacterial infection, diarrhoea and even some kinds of cancer, the question of whether we should try to eliminate it becomes much more finely balanced. It may be that the reason why the human body tolerates this bacterium is that, on the whole, the risks associated with infection by *H. pylori* are outweighed by the advantages. Perhaps stomach ulcers and gastric carcinoma are the price we pay to protect ourselves from a whole host of other conditions. The balancing act between one set of risks and another is often a difficult one, and the body can certainly get it wrong. But it would seem unwise to assume that medicine always knows best.

THE BENEFITS OF THE BLUES

Nothing illustrates the difficulty of determining whether or not a symptom is part of the solution or part of the problem than depression. Most doctors have assumed, not surprisingly, that depression is purely pathological, and have attempted to get rid of it by all manner of means, from drugs and various other kinds of physical therapy to counselling and psychoanalysis. A few people, however, have dared to suggest that the mental agony of melancholy might be just as protective as the physical pain to which it is often compared.

One of the most persuasive advocates of this view is Randolph Nesse, a psychiatrist at the University of Michigan School of Medicine. Nesse has argued that mood functions as an energy regulator, increasing levels of activity when the chances of success are high, and downshifting when times are lean. In Nesse's words, mood 'regulates the allocation of effort and resources – towards enterprises, strategies, and times likely to give a high payoff and away from unprofitable enterprises and times when efforts will likely be wasted or dangerous'.[16] Low mood, on this account, is triggered by a complex but largely unconscious estimation that action is futile or dangerous. The resulting loss of motivation leads a person to conserve his energy for more propitious times that may lie around the corner.

Nesse's theory may go some way to explaining the function of low mood, but this does not necessarily mean that it also accounts for depression. Whether or not it does depends on whether depression turns out to be simply an extreme version of low mood, or a wholly different syndrome. This question has dogged the debate about depression since the early days of modern psychiatry, and is still unresolved. Those who see depression as merely an extreme form of low mood can find some support for their view in the psychiatric manuals, which list 'low mood' as one of the core symptoms of the disorder; but to those who suffer from this condition, the mental torture can be so appalling that it seems to have little to do with what, in ordinary life, most people understand by this term. And, moreover, clinical depression is associated with a whole range of other symptoms that do not normally pop up when you just have the blues, such as sleep problems, bouts of anxiety and loss of appetite. It may be that while Nesse is right about the protective value of low mood, depression is something altogether different — a pathology rather than a defence.[17]

Even if we agree that depression is a pathology, and not an adaptive mechanism, the precise nature of what has gone wrong, and why, remains unclear. At present, all we have to go on are some suggestive clues emerging from research in comparative biology. The American primatologist Robert Sapolsky has studied the effects of social stress on wild baboons for many years. He has found that those at the bottom of the dominance hierarchy show many features also found in depressed humans. Levels of cortisol, for example, are dramatically elevated, while there is a corresponding decrease in levels of the neurotransmitter serotonin.[18]

Monkeys, apes and humans all derive great benefits from living in large groups, such as greater protection from predators, but there are also costs. In particular, living in bigger communities leads to increased competition with other members for resources, sexual partners and social rank. When they became highly social animals, then, primates struck a Faustian bargain, exchanging one kind of stress (predation) for another (social politics). In all primate groups, the stress is not distributed evenly across the social hierarchy: those at the bottom suffer more than those at the top. In such a situation, it may be counterproductive for those at the bottom of the pile to keep their stress mechanisms running — but that is, unfortunately perhaps, not an option. The physiological processes involved are not a detachable component that can be shed when one discovers that one is not the leader of the pack. They are deeply entrenched in our biology, the product of millions of years of evolution, and we are stuck with them whether we like it or not.

THE ORIGINS OF STRESS

The fight-flight response is something primates share not only with all other mammals, but all vertebrates. Indeed, the origins of this capacity go right back to the primitive defence mechanisms whose first appearance in sponges and molluscs we looked at briefly in the previous chapter. As it may be recalled, the immune systems of these simple animals function rather like perceptual systems, warning them of the presence of bacterial predators. Vertebrates, of course, receive information from many other sensory faculties besides the immune system. Most vertebrates have eyes that can see, ears that can hear, and noses that can detect smells. This gives mammals an advantage over molluscs when it comes to detecting predators. In addition to the predators that both molluscs and vertebrates can detect by means of their immune systems, which are generally far too small to be seen with the naked eye, and which do not emit sounds or smells, vertebrates can also see large, multicellular predators like lions and humans – and can spot them a long way off.

The challenge posed by these large predators was met by adapting the same physiological machinery that was already in place for dealing with the microscopic ones. This, at least, is what two American psychologists have argued. Steve Maier and Linda Watkins claim that the fight-flight response, which enables vertebrates to respond to large predators, evolved by co-opting the biological systems underlying the acute phase response that had already evolved, millions of years before.[19] In support of their claim, they point to the fact that both the innate immune response to infection and the fight-flight response to large predators activate the same immune-brain circuits. When a monkey or a human spots a lion moving rapidly towards them, for example, the hypothalamo-pituitary-adrenal (HPA) axis described in Chapter Three is activated, just as it is by IL-1 in the acute phase response. In both cases, the HPA axis responds with the same chemical cascade leading to the release of cortisol by the adrenal glands. This makes good sense, since cortisol breaks down the body's fat reserves into glucose that provides vital energy. Since both fighting and fleeing require rapid bursts of energy, and the machinery for generating such energy was already in place, natural selection simply wired the predator-detection mechanism up to the old HPA axis that had initially evolved for fighting infection.

Such conservatism is a common phenomenon in evolution. When a species is faced with a new problem that requires some evolutionary change, natural selection rarely goes back to the drawing board to design a completely new mechanism. Rather, it tends to co-opt some structure that is already there to serve some other function, and tinkers with it. The end result may not be perfect, but so long as it does the job, that is enough. Many apparently arbitrary features and design faults are only explicable in the light of this makeshift history. For example, it might seem odd that people get hot and sweaty when faced with a dangerous animal. Yet this psychological response is understandable in the light of the evolutionary history of the HPA axis. The HPA axis played a vital part in the acute phase response to infection long before it was co-opted in the service of the fight-flight response, and fever is — as we have already seen — an integral part of the acute phase response. The fact that fever is now also triggered by the sight of a dangerous animal is a by-product of this evolutionary legacy.

In fact, the tendency of the fight-flight response to activate processes that are designed more for fighting infection than for combating large animals may not be entirely without adaptive value. The risk of infection is increased when one is fleeing from, or engaging in combat with, another animal. Legs get scratched while running, and skin gets ripped when fighting.

Such breaks in the body's surface are obvious targets for bacterial invaders, so it may well be adaptive to prime the innate immune system for instant response on those occasions when wounds are more likely. The triggering of some of the features of the acute phase response by physical and psychological dangers may at first appear unrelated to infection, but it might in fact be a valuable anticipatory process, preparing the body for the increased risk of infection that attended such dangers in our evolutionary past.

For baboons at the bottom of the social hierarchy, the most immediate threat of injury may not be from a predator, but from the dominant baboons in the same troop. It may be quite adaptive, then, to be in a constant state of alert, the immune system continually primed by bursts of cortisol so that it can respond quickly to potential infections in the scratches caused by the surly alpha males. But, as with every biological adaptation, there are costs as well as benefits. The continual activation of the acute phase response can lead eventually to a state of chronic inflammation, in which sickness behaviour becomes a way of life. And this, perhaps, may be the closest we come in the animal world to a model of depression in humans. One important difference, of course, is that social hierarchies in human societies are not generally enforced by constant low-level physical assaults; the backbiting is metaphorical, not literal. But the biological effects may be very similar, leading to the same state of chronic activation of the acute phase response. Like low-status baboons, people at the bottom of the pile may find that their own defence mechanisms become the bane of their lives.

Chapter 7

THE ALTERNATIVES

There are many to whom the theory of toxic medicine will not appear at all new. A growing number of people in Europe and America are quite comfortable with the view that a certain kind of medicine, at least, has always tended to ride roughshod over the natural healing processes of the body. These people are linked by their search for alternative approaches to healing, approaches which they claim work with the body rather than against it.

The complementary and alternative medicine (CAM) movement embraces a wide range of systems.* Osteopathy, chiropractic, homeopathy, acupuncture, herbal medicine, spiritual healing and radionics are all quite different both in the techniques they use and in their theoretical assumptions. Their practitioners are united, however, by a common belief that their methods are much less toxic than the drugs and surgical procedures of orthodox Western medicine.

For some of the more fanatical believers, alternative medicine is completely safe, incapable of doing any damage whatsoever. The more realistic practitioners, however, admit that there are dangers. Potentially toxic concentrations of arsenic and

---

* The terms 'complementary medicine' and 'alternative medicine' are sometimes treated as if they referred to different things. In this book, I use them interchangeably to refer to a whole range of therapeutic practices that lie outside orthodox modern Western medicine.

cadmium have been found in homeopathic preparations, for example, and the use of unsterilised needles in acupuncture has led to the transmission of diseases such as HIV and hepatitis B.[1] Nevertheless, the risks associated with complementary medicine are probably less than those associated with orthodox medicine.

What about the other side of the equation, though? If the first law of pharmacology is true, the lower toxicity of alternative medicine should also mean that it is less effective. This, of course, is hotly disputed by the alternative therapists themselves. For them, it seems, the first law of pharmacology is something that only applies to conventional medicine. The pharmaceutical companies may be forced to make trade-offs between efficacy and toxicity, but no such dilemma faces the acupuncturist or the homeopath. In their minds, they have found the holy grail that eluded orthodox medicine – the remedy that is both effective and without side-effects.

THE EVIDENCE FOR ALTERNATIVE AND COMPLEMENTARY MEDICINE

The number of people using unorthodox therapies such as osteopathy, acupuncture and homeopathy grew rapidly in the 1980s and 1990s. In 1980, there were fewer than fourteen thousand practitioners of complementary medicine in the United Kingdom;[2] two decades later, the number had more than tripled.[3] Today, every high street has its health-food shop, and estimates suggest that by the late 1990s Americans were spending around $15 billion per year on complementary medicine.[4] Nor was the trend limited to grassroots support. By the year 2000, over half of British GPs had provided access to complementary medicine for their patients,[5] and a growing proportion of medical research funds in America and Europe was earmarked for investigating alternative therapies.

The last development has finally allowed the debate about complementary and alternative medicine to become more rational. During the 1980s, when alternative medicine was just beginning to grow in popularity, exchanges between orthodox doctors and alternative therapists were typically shrill and generated more heat than light. Homeopaths and herbalists caricatured mainstream medicine as narrow-minded, cold and oppressive, while doctors and surgeons dismissed the homeopaths as cranks and quacks. Neither side was able to base its claims on proper evidence, as the evidence was simply not there. Some critics suggested that the lack of evidence was itself a sinister ploy to undermine the credibility of alternative medicine, as the pharmaceutical companies which provided much of the funding for medical research clearly had no incentive to conduct clinical trials of remedies that they would not be able to patent.[6] Such conspiracy theories were overtaken by events, however, when the US Congress instructed the National Institutes of Health to research alternative medicine in 1992. Since then, a growing number of clinical trials of complementary and alternative therapies has allowed the claims and counter-claims to be assessed on the basis of proper scientific evidence.

So, what is the verdict? Does alternative medicine really work, or is it just a load of hogwash? This question does not admit of any simple answer. For one thing, as we have already noted, alternative medicine is an umbrella term that covers a dizzying variety of techniques and approaches. A report in 2000 by the British House of Lords Select Committee on Science and Technology distinguished almost thirty different disciplines, which ranged widely in the extent to which they can claim any scientific evidence in support of their claims.[7] Some, such as crystal therapy (in which various kinds of semi-precious stones are thought to possess healing properties) and iridology (which diagnoses disease by observing tiny flecks in the iris), have hardly been investigated, though their theories are so diametrically opposed to everything we know about physics and biology that it is probably not worth bothering to do so. Others, such as aromatherapy, have been subjected to some experimental investigation, but the results are at best mixed, and suggest that they are pure placebos. Finally, there is a small group of alternative therapies for which there is some evidence that, for certain medical conditions at least, they do work better than a placebo. This group includes osteopathy and chiropractic (both of which involve manipulating the body in various ways), herbal medicine and acupuncture.

Even with this group, the evidence is not very good. The clinical trials that have shown them to be more effective than placebos are often flawed. The most serious defect is probably the lack of proper blinding. Blinding means making sure that neither the patient nor the doctor knows whether a particular patient is receiving the experimental treatment or a placebo. This requires, among other things, that the placebo be indistinguishable from the active treatment in appearance, otherwise the blind can be 'broken', and patients and doctors can figure out who is getting the placebo and who isn't. If they can do this, the placebo response may occur in those given the experimental treatment, but not in those treated with the placebo. It would then appear as if the experimental treatment was better than a placebo, even if, in fact, it works entirely by evoking the placebo response.

For some kinds of alternative therapy, it is particularly difficult to ensure proper blinding. Acupuncture, for example, involves inserting needles into the skin at very precise points that supposedly correspond to certain 'meridians', or energy lines, that run throughout the body. Clearly, a sugar pill would not constitute a good placebo for testing acupuncture, as patients would know immediately who was getting the placebo and who was getting the experimental treatment. The most rigorous trials of acupuncture have used, as placebo, a 'sham' acupuncture treatment, in which needles are inserted into the skin just as in proper acupuncture, but not at the points corresponding to the supposed meridians. However, the person who carries out the sham acupuncture is typically a trained acupuncturist, who knows where the meridians are supposed to lie. Such studies cannot, therefore, be truly double-blind: the acupuncturist knows who is getting the experimental treatment and who is getting the placebo. And, as we have already seen, doctors give out subtle non-verbal cues that allow their patients to pick up on their degree of confidence in a treatment. There is, therefore, no such thing as a truly single-blinded study, where the doctor knows who is getting the placebo but the patient does not. As soon as the doctor knows, the patient does too – even if they might not be able to verbalise that knowledge.

The upshot of all this is that, even when clinical trials find that 'acupuncture does better than a placebo', the results should not be taken at face value. The difficulty of constructing a sham version acupuncture that is indistinguishable from the real thing means we can never be sure that acupuncture is anything more than a placebo, even when those receiving real acupuncture show more improvement than those receiving the sham version. It is also interesting to note that, in the few clinical trials that have found acupuncture to be 'better than a placebo', the patients were all suffering from conditions which we already know to be placebo-responsive. Trials of acupuncture for post-operative sickness and for easing neck and dental pain, for example, have found real acupuncture to outperform the sham version. When it comes to conditions that are not known to be placebo-responsive, such as recovery from stroke and osteo-arthritis, however, no difference has been found between acupuncture and placebo.[8] The most obvious explanation for this pattern is that blinding is not perfect in trials of acupuncture, allowing the placebo response to be activated more intensely by real acupuncture than by the sham version. The result is that acupuncture seems better than a placebo only when the condition being treated is, in fact, placebo-responsive. Acupuncture, in other words, is probably a pure placebo.

ARE CLINICAL TRIALS BIASED AGAINST ALTERNATIVE MEDICINE?

The difficulty of testing certain forms of alternative therapy has seemed to some to indicate a defect, not in the therapies themselves, but in the standard methods of scientific research.

If clinical trials cannot prove that acupuncture is better than a placebo, the argument goes, then there must be a problem with the methodology of clinical trials. Perhaps the effects of acupuncture and other alternative methods are too 'subtle' for the 'reductionist approach' of orthodox medical research.[9] Sometimes this argument takes on almost mystical overtones, in which the materialist approach of Western medicine is contrasted unfavourably with the spiritual sensitivity of the various alternatives. The clinical trial is then 'an essential tool for the mechanistic-objectifying paradigm' of orthodox medicine.[10]

The use, by those who take this view, of the term 'paradigm', borrowed from the philosopher Thomas Kuhn, suggests that alternative medicine has a completely different worldview, utterly incompatible with that of orthodox medicine. Andrew Vickers, of the Research Council for Complementary Medicine in London, has summarised this line of thought with admirable concision:

> There are two entirely separate paradigms, one associated with orthodox medicine and one with complementary medicine. Research methods are paradigm-specific, in other words, research methods used in one paradigm cannot be used in another. Therefore conventional research methodology is inappropriate for complementary medicine. Those working in a paradigm are unable to look outside of it. Conventional scientists are therefore blind to important healing phenomena.[11]

As Vickers points out, however, this argument is badly flawed. For one thing, the differences between different forms of alternative medicine are often greater than those between alternative medicine as a whole and mainstream medicine. It is therefore far too simplistic to regard complementary medicine as a single thing, opposed to an equally homogeneous orthodox approach. Even worse is the implication that people holding different views cannot engage in rational debate. Doctors and alternative therapists must simply agree to differ, because they work in different paradigms. Evidence and argument are completely abandoned.

Clearly, this is not a recipe for progress. If we wish to heal the rift between orthodox and complementary medicine, we must begin by finding some common ground, and the methodology of the clinical trial is the perfect candidate. Contrary to what some have claimed, the clinical trial is not 'biased' towards any particular school of thinking in medicine. It is grounded in very basic ideas about evidence that would, in any other context, hardly be open to dispute. When Ronald Fisher, one of the architects of modern statistics, offered a cup of tea to a woman standing next to him, she refused, remarking that she preferred the milk to be in the cup before the tea was added. Fisher thought this remark very silly, as he could not believe that it made any difference, whereupon the woman suggested an experiment. Immediately a trial was organised, and to Fisher's great surprise the woman identified more than enough cups of tea in which the tea had been poured first to prove that she could tell the difference. As this homely example illustrates, the principles of the clinical trial are really just common sense. Whether applied to tasting tea or testing medicine, they involve no special commitment to any particular 'paradigm'.

Ironically, the alternative therapists who reject the evidence of clinical trials on the grounds that this wonderfully neutral and objective method is irremediably biased succeed only in demonstrating their own biases. In his unfinished book *Snake Oil*, which recounts the various complementary therapies urged upon him by those who believed they could cure his terminal cancer, the journalist John Diamond tells the following story, which illustrates this point beautifully. Suppose someone offers to sell you a thousand chairs at the knockdown price of £10 each. You offer to write him a cheque, and he takes you into a massive room filled with chairs. 'There you are!' he says, 'a thousand chairs!' When you start to count them, he stops you. 'No need to count them,' he assures you, 'take my word for it; that's what a thousand chairs look like.' When you insist that you can't tell, just by looking, exactly how many chairs there are, and that counting is clearly the most logical and objective method for establishing their number, the chair-seller starts to get annoyed. 'I understand,' he says, 'that counting works pretty well in some circumstances, but it's a myth put about by self-serving mathematicians that it's the only way of assessing a number.'[12] The methodology of clinical trials is really no more than glorified counting. To accuse it of inherent bias is to reveal one's own.

HOMEOPATHY: A SPECIAL CASE

Homeopathy, n. A school of medicine midway between Allopathy and Christian Science. To the last both the others are distinctly inferior, for Christian Science will cure imaginary diseases, and they can not.

AMBROSE BIERCE, *The Devil's Dictionary* (1906)

Although some alternative therapies, such as acupuncture, present special problems when it comes to testing them, not all do. Homeopathic remedies, for example, are typically vials of colourless water, so indistinguishable placebos are not hard to produce. Unlike acupuncture, then, it is not hard to design trials of homeopathy in which there is proper double-blinding. This may explain, in part, why homeopathy is one of the most intensively studied forms of alternative medicine around. A meta-analysis of homeopathy published in the *Lancet* in 1997 found 186 controlled trials, of which over a hundred implemented all the standard methodological requirements such as randomisation and comparison with a placebo control group.[13] It seems that while a few practitioners of alternative therapies continue to reject the value of clinical trials, many are coming round to the idea that they represent a common standard by which both orthodox and complementary healing practices can be evaluated. Homeopaths, at least, do not seem afraid of submitting their techniques to scientific scrutiny.

So, does homeopathy work? After extensive statistical analysis, the 1997 *Lancet* study concluded that it is, on average, significantly more effective than a placebo. The study was accompanied by two independent commentaries commissioned by the *Lancet*, both of which cast doubt on the study. A subsequent letter to the *Lancet* complained that this showed that a double standard was at play here: when alternative therapies fail clinical trials, they are immediately dismissed as placebos, but when they pass, the trials themselves are impugned.[14]

At first sight, this attitude smacks of bias. It appears that a selective approach to the evidence of clinical trials, dismissing them whenever they do not give the results one wants, is not the exclusive preserve of alternative therapists, but can also be adopted by the defenders of scientific medicine when it suits their purposes. It is not, however, necessarily irrational to employ such a double standard. When an experiment yields a result that is perfectly compatible with everything else we know about the world, to reject it would certainly smack of dogmatism; but if the result conflicts with an entire corpus of well-established knowledge, it is sensible to treat it with some caution. It would be foolish indeed to cast aside the whole of physics, chemistry and biology – supported, as they are, by millions of experiments and observations – just because a single study yields a result that conflicts with their principles. And this is just what we would have to do if the result of the *Lancet* study were correct. For, to put it starkly, there is no place in our current scientific theories for any possible mechanism by which homeopathy might work, other than the placebo response. If homeopathy were really more effective than a placebo, therefore, we would have a major scientific revolution on our hands.

Homeopathy is rather special in this regard. There are many other forms of alternative medicine which, if they were shown to be more effective than a placebo, would not call for any great shift in scientific thinking. Herbalism is a case in point. Herbalists are only 'alternative' in the sense that the particular plants they use are not currently used by orthodox doctors. The basic idea of using plants to treat disease, however, is common to both alternative and orthodox medicine. About 70 per cent of pharmaceuticals now in use by orthodox doctors are, or derive from, natural plants.[15] Some remedies that were previously used only by alternative practitioners, such as St John's Wort, have since been shown to contain active ingredients that are more effective than a placebo for treating certain conditions, and are now regularly prescribed by orthodox physicians. But such discoveries do not undermine any of our current scientific theories. On the contrary, they lend even more weight to the basic idea that a drug can only be more effective than a placebo if it contains sufficient quantities of a biologically relevant chemical.

The incompatibility between homeopathy and current science lies not in the use of unorthodox herbs but in the use of ultra-high dilutions. Homeopaths believe that remedies retain biological activity – and even become more potent – if they are repeatedly diluted in water (and shaken between each dilution). Physics, however, allows us to calculate how many molecules of the active substance will remain in each sample of homeopathic remedy after each dilution. Some remedies that are sold as 'homeopathic' are not very dilute, and so may contain enough molecules of the original substance to warrant their description as herbal medicines rather than true homeopathic ones. In true 'classical' homeopathy, however, the remedies are diluted so many times that it is highly unlikely for most samples of the remedy to contain even one molecule of the active substance. Most homeopathic remedies are, in other words, pure water. And biology tells us that water is not a remedy for anything other than dehydration.

This line of argument assumes that the current theory of dilution is correct. According to the standard view, the molecules of a substance that is dissolved in water spread further and further apart as more water is added. In 2001, however, a team of chemists in South Korea found that some substances do not behave in this way.[16] Far from drifting further apart from each other when more water is added to the solution, the molecules of certain substances, such as DNA and even plain salt, actually clump together, first forming clusters of molecules, and then bigger aggregates of those clusters. These aggregates were typically five to ten times as big as those in the original solutions. This might provide a plausible rationale for the homeopathic practice of repeated dilution: perhaps larger aggregates may interact more easily with biological tissue. However, before homeopaths worldwide claim this discovery as the long-awaited scientific vindication of their work, a note of caution must be sounded. The solutions examined by the team in South Korea were only diluted five or six times, which is low by homeopathic standards, and certainly a long way from the ultra-high dilution that classical homeopathy is based on. Even if this discovery helps to explain why some low-dilution remedies may be effective, such remedies are better described as herbal medicines rather than homeopathic ones. True homeopathic remedies have been diluted so many times that the clustering mechanism is irrelevant; sheer numbers tell us that no molecules of the original substance will exist in most of them.

Some have gone to even greater lengths to square the principles of homeopathy with those of orthodox science. The French immunologist Jacques Benveniste, for example, has suggested that water has a kind of 'memory' that can retain information about the original substance that was added to it before the process of dilution.[17] This ghostly imprint is supposed to be more potent than the original substance itself. Such claims only make the conflict with science even more apparent, for there is no known physical or chemical mechanism that could plausibly serve as a basis for the hypothetical memory. Indeed, everything we know about the atomic and molecular structure of matter rules out such aquatic reminiscences. Still, this has not stopped Benveniste from going even further, and claiming that the memory of ultra-diluted water can be (1) erased by an alternating magnetic field, (2) transferred to 'naive' water by means of a specially configured amplifier, and (3) recorded on a computer hard disk and transmitted to 'naive' water over the Internet.[18] The discrepancy between the ideas of homeopathy and the established laws of physics is pushed to new heights here. Once again, we are faced with a stark choice: either homeopathy is simply a placebo, or the whole of physics and chemistry as we know them are false.

Since there is vastly more evidence in favour of current physics and chemistry than there is in favour of homeopathy, the most reasonable conclusion is that the *Lancet* study was somehow flawed. The doctors who wrote in to criticise it were not, therefore, guilty of hypocrisy. To be fair to the authors of the *Lancet* paper, it should be pointed out that their study was (unlike earlier experiments performed by Benveniste[19]) a model of methodological rigour, conforming to all the canons of ortho-dox medical research. It is not easy to see exactly where the flaws are. One possibility is that the quality of the trials was not in fact all that good. The authors of the study attempted to rebut this charge by showing that the superiority of homeopathy over placebo remained even when the analysis was restricted to the most rigorous trials. It was notable, however, that in this high-quality analysis the advantage of homeopathy over placebo was much reduced, and when such an adjustment removes much of the apparent effect, it is quite possible that what remains is due to residual bias and chance alone. Another possible flaw is that the results were distorted by publication bias. Clinical trials are much more likely to be published if they yield positive results, while negative results may be buried, so that a meta-analysis of published trials yields an artificially inflated estimate of efficacy. The authors of the *Lancet* study examined this possi-bility too, and argued that even if a certain degree of publication bias had occurred, it would not be enough to demolish their conclusions. Still, they did admit that 'although neither publi-cation bias nor poor-quality trials alone seem to explain our findings, we cannot be sure that combinations of these factors or others still unaccounted for might have led to an erroneous result'.

The whole affair illustrates beautifully just how complex, ambiguous and confusing is the process that we call scientific research. Despite their appearance of absolute impartiality and objectivity, even the most rigorous statistical analyses allow much scope for personal interpretation and subjective opinion. Far from putting a decisive end to the raucous squabbling of any healthy scientific discussion, it seems as if statistical methods merely allow disagreements to be more clearly stated in the language of numbers. There is, it seems, no way of circumventing the essentially chaotic process by which the scientific community settles important theoretical debates. And, even when a consensus is achieved, the verdict is never absolutely certain.

IT'S JUST A PLACEBO – BUT SO WHAT?

In the acrimonious wrangle over the results of the *Lancet* study on homeopathy, both sides failed to ask a fundamental question: what would it matter if homeopathy *were* pure placebo? The question can be extended to all the other forms of alternative medicine. Why does so much seem to hang on proving that they are more effective than a placebo? Beneath their differences, both supporters and critics of alternative medicine seem to agree that if it is shown to be no better than a placebo, then it is useless. Certainly, this was how one reviewer in the journal *Nature* summarised the results of a 2001 report showing that acupuncture was no more effective than a placebo for conditions other than some forms of sickness and pain: 'It is,' he concluded, 'virtually useless for the other conditions assessed.'[20]

Calling a treatment 'useless' suggests to my ears that people who are treated with it are no more likely to get better than those who remain untreated. This, however, is not the case with treatments that show no significant difference from a placebo. As we saw in Chapter Two, placebos are better than nothing when it comes to treating certain conditions such as pain, swelling and depression. People with these conditions who are treated with placebos are often substantially more likely to get better than those who are not treated at all. For Beecher, this was an amazing phenomenon, worthy of study in its own right. When he first observed that saline could produce similar effects to morphine, he was stunned. Nowadays, however, when the patients in the experimental arm of a clinical trial show the same recovery rate as those in the placebo arm, the reaction is not: 'Wow! The placebo works as well as the experimental drug!' It is: 'Oh dear! The drug is no better than a placebo.' No matter if the patients in both arms would have shown a massive improvement compared to a no-treatment group. That amazing phenomenon is completely ignored, because, as we have seen, a no-treatment group is rarely included.

We should also take into account the fact that consumer satisfaction among the users of complementary and alternative medicine tends to be very high. In 1993, when a group of midwives started prescribing lavender oil to women after child-birth – a practice recommended by aromatherapists for healing the perineum – they found that 85 per cent of the women felt the remedy had been of benefit.[21] When the same midwives subjected the treatment to a controlled clinical trial, they found no difference between real lavender oil and a synthetic lavender preparation.[22] The same mismatch between objective and subjective assessments of alternative medicine is found even when the patients themselves are asked for both kinds of evaluation. In one survey, for example, only 46 per cent of patients judged that a complementary therapy had *improved their condition greatly*, but 54 per cent said that they *felt much better* after visiting the practitioner. Clearly, an objective improvement in health is not the only thing that matters to patients.

This point upsets some doctors, who warn of the dangers of allowing good feelings to trump objective evidence of disease. To a certain extent, they are right. If someone goes to see an alternative practitioner, and comes away feeling happier even though his condition remains unchanged, he may be less likely to take further measures, and by the time the bad feelings come back it may be too late. Some of the less reputable alternative therapists have even been known to forbid their patients to consult orthodox doctors, although they have serious diseases such as cancer, and by the time these patients realise that the alternative therapy is not working, the cancer is too far advanced to be treated by conventional means either. To allow one's decisions about health to be dictated entirely by 'what feels best' is often clearly a disaster. However, this does not license the opposite conclusion, seemingly espoused by some doctors, that subjective feelings are completely irrelevant. Most people would not think it worth being kept alive if their condition condemned them to perpetual agony. Real-life decisions are usually not quite so black and white, but even in the case of a choice between a slightly more effective drug handed out by an uncaring doctor, and a less effective massage given by a caring aromatherapist, it is not clear that someone who chose the latter would necessarily be acting irrationally.

THE MEGA-PLACEBO EFFECT

The fact that consumer satisfaction is higher among users of alternative medicine than among those treated by conventional doctors raises the interesting possibility of what some have dubbed the 'mega-placebo effect'.[23] The idea is that, when it comes to treating conditions that are placebo-responsive, a pure placebo such as acupuncture might be more effective than a real treatment such as morphine. This may sound counter-intuitive, and it certainly challenges the traditional way of thinking about the placebo effect in clinical trials, so some explanation is called for.

When a drug is shown to be more effective than a placebo in a clinical trial, it is important to remember that this result applies to a particular kind of placebo. To be precise, we should say that such drugs have been shown to be more effective than *placebos that are identical in shape, size and so on*. The placebo response in each arm of the trial is artificially equalised by the process of double-blinding which, when done properly, ensures that there is no room for any difference in the degree of belief invested in either treatment. They look, taste and feel exactly the same.

It cannot, however, be inferred from this that clinically proven drugs will always be more effective than every kind of placebo in every context. We have already seen that placebo responses can vary enormously, depending on the degree of belief that the patient has in the treatment he is receiving. The specific effect of a drug, on the other hand, is likely to be much less variable. This means that, when it comes to treating placebo-responsive conditions such as pain and depression, the variation in the overall effect of a treatment will depend much more on the size of the placebo response it evokes than on the size of the specific effect.

An analogy might help to make this point clearer. When it comes to placebo-responsive conditions, the total effect of an active treatment is rather like the length of a concertina. The length of a concertina comprises both a fixed measurement for each handle, and a variable one for the middle bit that can stretch and be compressed. In the same way, the total effect of an active drug used to treat a placebo-responsive condition comprises both a fixed amount for the specific effect, and a variable amount for the placebo response. A pure placebo is like a concertina with no handles. In clinical trials, the middle bit of each concertina is kept fixed, so that the size of the handles can be measured by subtracting the length of the concertina without handles from the length of the concertina with handles. But in real life, no such restriction is imposed. The concertina can be stretched and squashed wildly from one context to another.

It is perfectly possible, then, for the concertina with no handles to be longer, overall, than the concertina with handles. If the former is stretched to its maximum length, and the latter is squashed as much as possible, the difference might be very great. This is the idea of the mega-placebo effect. A pure placebo, such as acupuncture, could be more effective in treating placebo-responsive conditions than a real drug if patients had much more faith in the placebo than in the drug.

TIME AND RITUAL

The existence of the mega-placebo effect is, at the moment, only a theoretical possibility, and has never been demonstrated in reality. That, however, may simply be because nobody has ever really *attempted* to demonstrate it. The difficulties of constructing a good way of investigating the phenomenon, together with the lack of funding for this kind of study (which would certainly not please the big pharmaceutical companies), have hampered investigation in this area. Nevertheless, there are some grounds for thinking that the mega-placebo effect may be widespread.

Chief among these is the rapidly growing popularity of alternative medicine, which is correlated with an increasing sense of disillusionment with orthodox medicine. The high levels of consumer satisfaction among users of alternative medicine suggest that alternative therapists are better at evoking confidence and trust in their patients, and so better able to mobilise the placebo response, than are conventional doctors. A whole host of factors are probably responsible for this, not least of which is the fact that alternative therapists can devote more time to each patient. The average length of time an alternative therapist spends with a patient is around forty minutes, while the current pressures on GPs to maximise efficiency mean that they cannot afford to be so liberal. In 1943 the average time that American GPs spent with each patient was twenty-six minutes; in 1985 it was down to seventeen minutes.[24] Today it is even less – some estimates put it as low as six minutes.

Another factor is the enthusiasm and faith of the doctor himself. Alternative therapists are typically great believers in their systems. Unlike orthodox doctors, whose training is paid for by the government in many countries, alternative practitioners must generally pay for their own training; they would probably not undertake such a risk if they did not have a high degree of belief in their particular type of therapy prior to the training. Orthodox doctors, on the other hand, are not required to be especially committed to any particular kind of treatment. Quite the opposite, in fact: organised scepticism is an essential part of the training in scientific medicine. We have already seen how doctors and therapists communicate their expectations of success to their patients through subtle non-verbal cues of which they themselves may be completely unaware. This could have a big impact on the effectiveness of treatments used for placebo-responsive conditions.

Closely related to the belief in the efficacy of the treatment itself is the manner in which it is given. Alternative therapists often surround the administration of their remedies with a certain degree of ritual. Orthodox doctors, on the other hand, tend to write out prescriptions to their patients in a routine way, without any fanfare. The distinguished Canadian essayist and novelist Robertson Davies described the negative effect of this increasingly technical approach to administering drugs:

> When I was a boy, [the] doctor . . . examined me gravely, asked questions that were searching [, and] retired . . . [He] emerged with a bottle from which he instructed me to drink three times a day . . . I regarded the doctor as a magician . . . [In my] adult life my various doctors have given me medicine – it tends to be in pill form nowadays – which plainly comes from a pharmaceutical company, and I leave his office thinking of him as a middleman between me and a large pill works. He has lost his magic.[25]

HEALING WITH HANDS

In their fascinating book *Magic or Medicine?*, Richard Buckman and Karl Sabbagh cite several other changes that have eroded the placebo effect in conventional medicine. In particular, they draw attention to the increasing physical distance between doctor and patient that has accompanied the rise of medical technology. Nowadays, diagnosis is often accomplished by means of x-rays and scans, and therapeutic procedures that do involve contact, such as surgery, are often carried out while the patient is unconscious or anaesthetised. Many alternative practitioners, on the other hand, engage in direct physical contact with their patients. Acupuncture, chiropractic and osteopathy all involve extensive contact, both in diagnosing the problem and in treating it. An osteopath, for example, will tap, touch and prod different areas of the patient's body to build up a picture of what is wrong, before manipulating various joints to correct the problem.

According to Patrick Wall, whose ideas we looked at in Chapter Five, natural selection has designed specific brain circuits to feed information about the social environment into the circuits that control the feeling of pain. It is possible that these circuits use the feeling of being touched as an indicator of social support. Certainly, chimpanzees − our closest living relatives − use touch in this way. They spend hours each day grooming each other, picking ticks off each other's backs. This is far more than a hygienic measure: it is an important signal of social support. If a chimpanzee is attacked by another member of the group, he is far more likely to receive help from a grooming partner than from anyone else. Grooming is part of the social cement that holds together the friendships and alliances that are so vital to life in a troop of chimps.

Whatever its evolutionary origins may be, the power of touch has long been exploited by humans for therapeutic purposes. Massage is one of the oldest medical practices on record: it was practised in ancient Egypt, and Hippocrates recommended that doctors should 'be experienced in many things, but assuredly in rubbing'. Current medical thinking attributes the benefit of massage to the direct physical action on the muscles themselves, but it is quite possible that much of it is due rather to the fact that being touched by another is interpreted by the brain as a signal of social support. This interpretation is bolstered by the finding, in the study of the effects of fake ultrasound, that the benefits of being massaged with the switched-off ultrasound applicator were only felt when the massage was given by someone else.

Between the beginning of the fourteenth century and the beginning of the nineteenth, thousands of people in Europe visited their monarchs for the 'royal touch', a ceremony in which the king would lay his hands upon the sick. The most common condition for which people would seek this kind of help was 'scrofula' – also known as 'the King's Evil' – a vague term that probably covered a variety of different problems. The main symptoms were swellings and ulcers around the face and neck, which have been attributed by modern medical authorities to tuberculosis of the lymph nodes, but many cases may have been due to other causes, such as chaffing and repetitive strain.

History does not record the precise success rate of the royal therapy in healing scrofulous subjects, and it may well have had no effect at all. Certainly, 'the laying on of hands' is a common trick that has been used by many quacks and frauds, from the notorious Valentine Greatraks, also known as 'the Stroker', who conned money out of gullible sick people in seventeenth-century England, to the equally fraudulent Christian 'healers' who practise similar tricks in America today.[26] Given all we have said about the power of touch to evoke and enhance the placebo response, however, it is interesting to note that all the conditions diagnosed as scrofula involve a pronounced inflammatory component. If, as I have been arguing, the placebo response is simply the suppression of the inflammatory response, it is quite possible that the royal touch did produce some symptomatic relief, even if it was powerless to cure the tuberculosis that probably underlay many cases of scrofula. At the very least, the popularity of this practice – King Charles I alone is said to have touched some 100,000 sick people – suggests an instinctive awareness that touch can be a powerful therapeutic agent.

SEPARATING THE WHEAT FROM THE CHAFF

Unconventional treatments often seem to make people feel more comfortable, even when their accompanying theories are silly.

EDWARD W CAMPION, *New England Journal of Medicine*
(1993)

The various ingredients which distinguish the typical consultation with a conventional doctor from one with an alternative therapist – such as time, enthusiasm, ritual and touch – are all likely to enhance the placebo response in alternative therapy and diminish it in conventional medicine. This effect will only occur when treating placebo responsive conditions, of course, but there is evidence that the majority of consultations with alternative therapists are for things like back pain and stress-related conditions – in other words, for just those phenomena that we know respond to placebos.

It is therefore quite possible that, in the context of actual clinical practice, certain kinds of alternative therapy may be more effective than orthodox medicine at relieving certain conditions, even though they are pure placebos. This mega-placebo effect could be investigated by instigating more of the so-called 'pragmatic' clinical trials. These differ from the standard placebo-controlled randomised clinical trials in that they generally compare two therapies that are both believed to be active, rather than one active therapy with a placebo, and also allow each arm of the trial to work in 'optimal' circumstances, rather than forcing them to conform to artificially standardised conditions. While this kind of clinical trial is much less 'clean' than a standard trial, and raises all sorts of methodological and statistical difficulties, these disadvantages may be outweighed by the advantage of greater realism.

Pragmatic clinical trials comparing an alternative therapy with an orthodox treatment would tell us which is more effective in the real world, but they would not help to answer the question of whether alternative therapies work entirely by means of the placebo effect. For many people, however, this question may be rather academic. What does it matter, they may ask, if an alternative therapy is just a placebo, so long as it works? From a purely therapeutic point of view, of course, it doesn't. But from a scientific one, it certainly does matter.

Many alternative therapies are not presented simply as therapeutic techniques, but rather come bundled up with a particular theory as to how the technique works. The needling technique of acupuncture, for example, is often (though not always) taught alongside the theories of traditional Chinese medicine, according to which a special kind of energy known as 'qi' flows along channels known as meridians. The art of prescribing homeopathic remedies is taught alongside the strange ideas discussed earlier, such as the principle of dilution and the 'memory' of water. As already noted, these bizarre notions are completely at odds with everything we know about physics, chemistry and biology. Despite hundreds of years of anatomical dissection and decades of microbiology, nobody has ever once observed a meridian or measured a quantum of qi. And, despite claims to the contrary, nobody has ever succeeded in recording the memory of water on a computer's hard disk.

It is the association of alternative therapies with these crackpot theories that is responsible for the continuing schism between orthodox and complementary medicine. If the techniques of alternative medicine could be separated from the dubious theories that sometimes accompany them, the way would be open to a much more profound dialogue between orthodox and complementary practitioners, and a greater integration of conventional and complementary healthcare. There is always the possibility, of course, that doing away with the crackpot theories that provide alternative therapies with some of their appeal might actually rob them of their effectiveness, by destroying the vital belief that enables them to mobilise the placebo response. In such cases, we face a choice of a clearly ethical nature: to preserve the effectiveness of these therapies by perpetuating crazy theories, or to seek the truth at the risk of robbing some patients of their favourite therapeutic resources. I deal with such thorny ethical problems in Chapter Nine. For the time being, the important point is that the search for the truth about healing need not lead us to throw out the baby of alternative techniques with the bathwater of alternative medical theories. The key to a fruitful dialogue between orthodox and alternative medicine would be for all concerned to recognise that evoking the placebo response is itself a legitimate therapeutic activity.

If the placebo response comes to be seen as a valuable therapeutic resource rather than as mere noise that interferes with the measurement of specific effects, alternative practitioners might be happier to give up their specious claims about energy fields and auras, and accept the idea that their therapies are powerful placebos. And if orthodox practitioners recognise the value of evoking the placebo response as an adjunct to all the specific effects of the various drugs at their disposal, they might be more inclined to learn a few lessons from the way alternative practitioners treat their patients, instead of dismissing them as quacks. Doctors might then discover how to regain the magic they have lost, and research into the placebo response could allow medicine to heal itself.

Chapter 8

PSYCHOTHERAPY — THE PUREST PLACEBO?

For those who are fortunate enough never to have experienced a panic attack, it is hard to convey an idea of the sheer terror that sweeps over the sufferer. Without warning, the heart starts beating madly, the hands start shaking uncontrollably, and beads of sweat well up on the face. Breathing may become harder, sometimes leading to a feeling that one is being choked, and there may be chest pain and feelings of dizziness. A sense of impending doom and a fear of going crazy — or even dying — grip the mind, leading to a desperate urge to escape, to be anywhere except *here*.

In the mid-1990s, while working as a psychotherapist in a clinical psychology department in London, I was charged with treating a middle-aged man whose panic attacks were not responding to medication. Despite taking three times the recommended daily dose of beta-blockers, which he supplemented with liberal amounts of the oldest anti-anxiety drug known to man — alcohol — my patient was still having one or two attacks every day. After several weeks of therapy, I could still see no pattern to the attacks, but one day it dawned on me that they always occurred when the man *had to write something in public*. One attack, for example, took place when he had to sign his name in the visitors' book at the reception of an office where he had an appointment; another when he had to write something on a board for others to see.

At the time, I was under the influence of psychoanalytic

theory, and looked for some repressed desire that would explain why this particular situation had become the trigger for the man's attacks. I soon found one. He had been an avid writer in his spare time, sending out manuscripts to publishers left, right and centre, until repeated rejections finally crushed his spirit, and he gave up his scribbling. When I pointed out the connection between the abandoned wish and the trigger for the panic attacks, the man was convinced that we had got to the bottom of his problem. And, sure enough, when he returned the following week, he was able to report that the attacks had completely vanished. Over the following four weeks, he only had one more attack, despite reducing his alcohol intake and ceasing to take the beta-blockers altogether. A well-timed psychoanalytic interpretation, it seemed, had accomplished what medication could not.

Or had it? The usual caveats about individual case-histories must be borne in mind here. Perhaps the fact that the man's symptoms abated the week after I offered my psychoanalytic interpretation was pure coincidence. And, even if there was some causal link between the interpretation and the remission of symptoms, this might have been due entirely to the placebo effect. In other words, the interpretation I offered, linking the man's abandoned wish to be a writer with the trigger for his attacks, may have been factually incorrect as an explanation of the symptom; perhaps the interpretation only caused the attacks to cease because the man *believed* it would. To investigate these possibilities, we need to turn to clinical trials and statistical research. We should not let the power of narrative put our critical faculties to sleep.

PUTTING PSYCHOTHERAPY TO THE TEST

Before we ask whether the benefits of psychotherapy are due to the placebo effect, we should first pause to ask whether psychotherapy does, in fact, produce any benefit at all. This is a fraught area of discussion, and there is still no consensus as to what the answer is. For a long time, there were no real data either way.

Various types of psychotherapy flourished for half a century before anybody bothered to subject them to rigorous clinical evaluation. Freud invented psychoanalysis, the first 'talking cure', at the end of the nineteenth century, and in the first few decades of the twentieth century it spawned a dozen or so variants – Jungian analysis, Adlerian therapy, Kleinian analysis and other such creatures. By the middle of the century, psychotherapy had conquered America, and had also become very influential in Britain and France. Then, in 1952, a young German psychologist working in Britain published a pioneering study of the effects of psychotherapy. Hans Eysenck, who was also to become famous for his work on IQ, compared the improvement rate in 7293 people undergoing psychotherapy with that of a control group who had similar neurotic problems but had received no psychotherapy. The results were damning. Of those receiving psychotherapy, 64 per cent had improved; but in the control group 72 per cent had made a recovery within two years of their breakdown without any psychotherapeutic assistance.[1]

Eysenck concluded that 'roughly two-thirds of a group of neurotic patients will recover or improve to a marked extent within two years of the onset of their illness, whether they are treated by means of psychotherapy or not'. In other words, psychotherapy was completely powerless to relieve neurosis. As far as neurotic symptoms are concerned, it made no difference whether or not you went to see a psychotherapist.

Naturally, Eysenck's study aroused intense reactions in the psychotherapeutic community. Some responded with obscurantism, rejecting the very attempt to evaluate psychoanalysis by 'crude' statistical methods and asserting the superiority of individual intuition above objective evidence, an attitude summed up in the following excerpt from the *American Handbook of Psychiatry*:

For the patient, his immediate knowledge of the effect of analysis is sufficient evidence of its worth, however sceptical the outside observer may be and however lacking the statistics to 'prove' its usefulness. Perhaps its effectiveness can never be shown by scientific methods . . . Perhaps the experience of analysis is like that of beauty, of mysticism, of love – self-evident and world-shaking to him who knows it, but quite incommunicable to another who does not.[2]

This dogmatic assertion of the value of psychoanalysis, together with the refusal to consider the possibility that any evidence at all could ever undermine it, has more in common with religious faith than with the balanced pursuit of truth. It is clearly not a recipe for rational debate. Not everyone in the psychotherapeutic community has buried his head in the sand, however. Some have taken up the challenge posed by Eysenck's initial study, and attempted to meet him on the firm ground of scientific evidence.

It took these more scientifically-minded psychotherapists twenty-five years to mount a sufficiently powerful rejoinder to Eysenck's blistering attack. In 1977, the *American Psychologist* published a meta-analysis summarising the results of hundreds of 'outcome studies' – the psychotherapists' equivalent of clinical trials.[3] After criticising earlier studies, such as Eysenck's, on the grounds that their methods were inadequate for making sense of the complex data, the two authors, M.L. Smith and Gene Glass, concluded that patients receiving psychotherapy were significantly more likely to get better than those who do not receive it.

IS PSYCHOTHERAPY JUST A PLACEBO?

Needless to say, the 1977 meta-analysis did not put an end to the controversy. The critics of psychotherapy were quick to point out that it had several major flaws, not least of which was the grouping together and equal weighting of studies of very diverse quality. Another serious problem was that the meta-analysis pooled the results of studies that investigated many different kinds of psychotherapy for many different kinds of condition. The most serious problem of all, however, was that very few of the studies included in the meta-analysis bothered to include a placebo control group. Most simply compared the recovery rate of patients undergoing a form of therapy with that of patients who were not receiving therapy (but who were on a waiting list). Even if one accepts the conclusion that psychotherapy is beneficial, then, the possibility remains that the benefits of psychotherapy are due entirely to the placebo effect.

To their credit, the authors of the 1977 meta-analysis did attempt to answer this question. In a subsequent book based on the same set of studies, Smith and Glass estimated that half of the beneficial effects of psychotherapy were due to the placebo effect.[4] In other words, psychotherapy was twice as effective as a placebo. When another group of researchers re-analysed the same data, they arrived at the same numerical result.[5] They interpreted this result in a rather different way, however. Instead of concluding, as Smith and Glass had done, that psychotherapy was more than just a placebo, the second group argued for exactly the opposite conclusion.

This disagreement is instructive. It is further warning, if any were needed, that numbers do not speak for themselves. The mere fact that the studies examined by Smith and Glass show psychotherapy to be more effective than the various placebo controls that were used does not prove that psychotherapy is in fact more than a placebo. To see why not, it is necessary to look at the kind of placebos to which the various forms of psychotherapy have been compared.

Here, of course, we immediately run into the same difficulty that we encountered when looking at clinical trials of acupuncture: what would count as a proper placebo in this context? A proper placebo is one that neither the patient nor the doctor can tell apart from the 'real thing'. If the patients or the doctors involved in a clinical trial can guess who is getting the placebo and who is getting the real thing, the belief effect might work just for those who are getting the real thing. Even if the real thing was itself a pure placebo, it would outperform the placebo in the trial simply because it was *a more believable placebo*, and we might conclude, mistakenly, that it was more than just a placebo. Some placebos are more powerful than others.

This problem affects every one of the few trials in Smith and Glass's study that compared psychotherapy with a placebo. The 'placebos' used in these trials ranged from listening to records or stories and muscle relaxation training to group discussions and even sugar pills. It would have been immediately obvious to everyone involved in the trials who was getting psychotherapy and who wasn't. If there was a general belief in the power of psychotherapy among the participants, any positive results in favour of psychotherapy might well be due to that *belief* rather than to the techniques of psychotherapy *per se*. Even if the people involved had no particular beliefs about the effectiveness of psychotherapy, the sheer length of time that even a brief course of therapy takes might have caused them to believe that they were getting a more powerful treatment than they would from a mere pill. To really show that psychotherapy is more than just a particularly powerful placebo, it is necessary to control for these other confounding factors.

Fortunately, a few studies have attempted to provide credible 'dummy therapies' that are not obviously distinguishable from the real thing. In one famous experiment conducted in 1979 by Hans Strupp and Suzanne Hadley, for example, one group of fifteen patients suffering from depression or anxiety was treated by trained and experienced psychotherapists, while a comparable patient group was treated by university professors with no psychological training at all. At the end of the study, the patients treated by the university professors showed as much improvement as those treated by the psychotherapists.[6] Several other studies have also found that there is no significant difference in outcomes whether therapy is provided by experienced professionals or by inexperienced non-professionals.[7]

The fact that years of practical and theoretical training make little if any difference to the benefit provided by psychotherapy is not conclusive proof that it is a pure placebo, but it does point very strongly in that direction. The scales are tipped even further that way by the repeated finding that different types of psychotherapy (verbal or behavioural, psychoanalytic or cognitive, and so on) do not produce noticeably different types or degrees of benefit.[8] If the vast differences of methodology and technique between the various types of psychotherapy have no impact on recovery, then it seems plausible that the benefits of psychotherapy are due entirely to the one thing that all these different approaches have in common – the cultivation of the belief in the patient that he or she is receiving *bona fide* medical help.

WOULD IT MATTER IF PSYCHOTHERAPY WAS PURE PLACEBO?

The idea that psychotherapy may be a pure placebo – that it only works to the extent that those receiving it believe it will help them – has been greeted with joy by the critics of psychotherapy and with alarm by many therapists. Both sides assume that this finding, if it were established, would deal a deadly blow to the practice of psychotherapy. According to one outspoken critic of psychotherapy, for example, the placebo charge is fatal:

> Proof that psychotherapy adds little to common human kindness or to simple social activities – that it does not build on placebo responses and that it may in essence be little more than a placebo response – invalidates the professional utility of the field.[9]

Others, however, take a rather different view of the matter. The medical anthropologist Arthur Kleinman argues that to describe psychotherapy as a pure placebo is to pay therapists a compliment, not to insult them:

Psychotherapy may very well be a way of maximising placebo responses . . . but if so, it should be applauded, rather than condemned, for exploiting a useful therapeutic process which is underutilised in general health care.[10]

To some extent, Kleinman is right. If you are simply interested in whether psychotherapy can benefit people with certain conditions, it shouldn't matter too much whether it is a placebo or not. Placebos can alleviate some conditions, including some of the main conditions for which psychotherapy is typically used, such as depression and anxiety, and some people would rather cure their ills by talking to a therapist than by taking a pill. For these people, psychotherapy may be the best method; there may even be a mega-placebo effect, similar to that which may be at work in some cases of alternative therapy. Those who believe that psychotherapy works may endow it with a greater placebo effect than that which attaches to the pills handed out by an unsympathetic doctor, with the result that the pure placebo is more effective than an active drug.

This is mere speculation, however. Nobody has ever produced any evidence that mega-placebo effects really exist. In fact, the relatively small difference in the effects of sugar pills and 'placebo therapies' suggests that sugar pills can be just as powerful as more elaborate placebos such as intensive psychotherapy. It would be interesting to see whether more psychotherapeutically-minded people get more out of a placebo therapy than a placebo pill, but this experiment has never been done. There is, however, some reason to doubt that such an experiment would vindicate Kleinman's rosy view of psychotherapy.

Kleinman suggests that, even if psychotherapy is a pure placebo, this would not necessarily threaten the livelihood of psychotherapists, since good therapists might excel at the art of evoking the placebo effect. They might even have a few things to teach the medical profession, so that doctors could become better at eliciting placebo responses in their patients.

Unfortunately for Kleinman, however, the study by Strupp and Hadley rather undermines this idea. The fact that patients treated by trained and experienced psychotherapists fare no better than those treated by university professors with no psychological training at all does not bode well for the idea that therapists have great secrets to impart to the medical profession.

A PANOPLY OF THEORIES

Most therapists do not share Kleinman's optimism. For them, the discovery that most – if not all – forms of psychotherapy are pure placebos would undermine their whole profession. Their fears seem well-founded, since there is one obvious way in which such a discovery would indeed pull the rug from under their feet: it would, in one fell swoop, invalidate the whole panoply of theories that purport to justify the various techniques that make each style of psychotherapy distinct from the others.

As we have already seen, the term 'psychotherapy' covers a wide range of approaches. The amazing variety of clinical techniques that go under this banner is underpinned by an equally diverse range of theories, each of which is supposed to legitimise a given technique. Freudian psychoanalysts offer their patients interpretations of repressed wishes because, according to the Freudian theory of the mind, this technical procedure should lead to a lifting of neurotic symptoms. Behavioural thera-pists use very different methods, such as desensitisation (which we will examine shortly), because they subscribe to a different theory of how the mind works. Each school of psychotherapy has its own pet theory to justify and explain why its particular clinical techniques should work.

Not one of these various theories, however, claims that psychotherapy works by means of the placebo effect. No school of psychotherapy claims that its favoured clinical techniques are effective only because, and only to the extent that, the patients *believe* them to be effective. Such an idea has, in fact, always been anathema, ever since Freud first opposed psychoanalysis to hypnotism and other forms of 'suggestion'. 'Suggestion' was never properly defined by Freud or his followers, but came to be a vague pejorative term that members of rival schools could throw at each other. The term 'placebo', too, has often been used in this way, as a term of insult exchanged between members of rival therapeutic schools. Howard Brody, a professor of medicine at Michigan State University, recounts the story of two Korean acupuncturists who met at a conference. They had been getting on quite well until they discovered that each practised a slightly different style of acupuncture. Immediately, each accused the other of purveying a placebo.[11]

Kleinman would no doubt think that these two acupuncturists were naive, since in his view there is nothing wrong with purveying a placebo; but that would be to miss the point. There may be nothing wrong with purveying a placebo if that is all you are claiming to do, but most practitioners of alternative medicine, along with the vast majority of psychotherapists, claim precisely the opposite. They assert that their techniques work because the mind, or the body, is organised in such-and-such a way. If the efficacy of such techniques turned out to depend simply on whether or not the patient *believes* in them, this would cast serious doubt on the underlying theories. And, if it becomes generally known that these therapies are based on false theories, they will probably lose any therapeutic power they may currently have. Placebos only work to the extent that patients believe in them, and the theories that underwrite the various forms of alternative medicine and psychotherapy play a large part in fostering that belief. It would be naive, then, to think that alternative therapists and psychotherapists could go on practising their various techniques if it became generally known that they were mere placebos. Such a discovery would rob these placebos of their placebogenic powers.

THE THEORY OF REPRESSION

Take the case of my panic-stricken patient, for example, whose cure I related at the beginning of this chapter. The fact that his panic attacks cleared up so quickly after I had offered him my psychoanalytic interpretation – pointing out the connection between the trigger for his attacks and his repressed wish to be a writer – might well be just a coincidence. But if it was not – if the interpretation really caused the panic attacks to disappear – that still leaves open the question of *how* it did this. One possibility is that the interpretation happened to be right, and allowed the patient to bring his repressed wish into the bright light of consciousness, where it lost its pathogenic powers. Another possibility is that the interpretation was wrong – either because the symptom was caused by a different repressed wish, or because the whole theory of repression itself is false – but that it activated the placebo response because the patient *believed* the interpretation was therapeutic.

Freud did not deny that the second kind of process could happen, but he vigorously denied that real psychoanalysis worked in this way. Psychoanalysis, he argued, worked whether the patient believed in it or not, and this was what distinguished it from suggestion – his term for hypnotherapy. Freud thought that suggestion and hypnotherapy worked by implanting certain kinds of belief in the patient's mind, beliefs which could then trigger the healing process. In other words, they were pure placebos. And, of course, psychoanalysis was supposed to be much more effective than mere suggestion. A cure produced by suggestion would, Freud claimed, be short-lived; only psychoanalysis could rid the patient of his symptom once and for all. When some of his early followers – first Jung, then Adler – broke away from the Freudian orthodoxy and set up their own schools of therapy, Freud was therefore able to explain their therapeutic successes while at the same time derogating them. Unlike the original Freudian-style psychoanalysis, he claimed, Jungian analysis and Adlerian therapy worked by suggestion – they were placebos, producing cures even though the interpretations offered by the therapists were false, simply because the patients were gullible. In the long run, the patients would surely relapse, unlike those who had been treated by strictly Freudian methods.

Unfortunately for Freud, this argument soon began to backfire, hoisting him by his own petard. For one thing, it soon became apparent that his own patients were just as likely to relapse as those treated by heretics like Jung and Adler. And, worse, the Freudian church itself became so broad that, even when two analysts both called themselves Freudians, they would be likely to differ on important points of doctrine. By Freud's own reasoning, then, the practice of suggestion had to be endemic among his most faithful disciples as well as among the heretics, a point noted by one of his English followers, Edward Glover:

> . . . when psychoanalysts differ on important points of doctrine, one or other of the contesting parties must, however unwillingly, be practising suggestion on his patients instead of analysing them.[12]

As there did not seem to be any clear superiority of one kind of psychoanalysis over any other, the logical conclusion was that it was not simply 'one or the other' who was practising suggestion, but that *all* analysts were.[13] The possibility that psychoanalysis was, in the end, pure placebo, haunted Freud throughout his life, and though he sought long and hard for a way of proving the contrary, he never succeeded.

BEHAVIOUR THERAPY

By the 1970s, the handful of Freudian-type therapies that had arisen in the early decades of the twentieth century had sprouted many more offshoots, some of which no longer had much in common with their distant ancestors. Perhaps the most important distinction to be drawn amongst the plethora of competing approaches is that between the so-called 'insight' or 'verbal' therapies, and the more 'cognitive' or 'behavioural' methods. The insight therapies, which included the original psychoanalytic method invented by Freud, aimed to cure neurotic disorders by revealing to the patient the hidden truths buried in his own mind. The more modern cognitive and behavioural methods, which were mostly developed in the 1960s, eschewed this lofty ambition for the more down-to-earth objective of training the patient to adopt different habits of thought and new patterns of behaviour.

These modern therapies rely on very different theories about how the mind works, theories that are currently believed to have much more scientific value than the various hypotheses entertained by Freud and his followers. One form of behaviour therapy, for example, known as desensitisation or 'exposure therapy', is based on the phenomenon of conditioning. As we have already seen, conditioning is a well-established psychological process in which an animal learns to produce a response to a stimulus that would not normally elicit that response. Pavlov's dogs, for example, learned to salivate in response to the sound of a bell ringing.

Desensitisation is an attempt to press the process of conditioning into the service of psychotherapy for various kinds of phobia. The idea is relatively straightforward. Just as Pavlov's dogs learned to associate the sound of a bell with the arrival of food, so phobic people must have learned to associate the phobic stimulus (such as a spider for arachnophobics, or being in a public place for agoraphobics) with the arrival of danger. To eliminate this fear, the behaviour therapist attempts to instil the opposite association: the phobic patient must be taught to associate the stimulus with the *absence* of danger. Various methods are used in pursuit of this goal. For example, an arachnophobic might be encouraged to handle, first a plastic spider, and eventually a real one, in the hope that repeated exposure to the stimulus in the absence of any real danger will eventually lead the patient to perceive spiders as harmless.

Several studies have shown desensitisation to be a reasonably effective way of combating phobias. Few, however, have asked whether the method works by virtue of the conditioning process just described, or whether in fact it is just another example of the placebo effect, and works simply because patients believe it does. One or two studies, though, suggest that there may indeed be a large placebo element in desensitisation therapy. One group, for example, compared desensitisation therapy for people who were scared of either spiders or snakes with an elaborate placebo therapy.[14] The patients in the placebo group were told that they would be viewing pictures of spiders or snakes, but that these would be flashed on a screen too rapidly for the conscious mind to perceive. They were further informed that the pictures would be perceived subliminally, and any phobic responses elicited by them would be recorded and would trigger the delivery of a mild electric shock to their fingers. The rationale for this procedure was explained in terms of conditioning.

In fact, the patients were not shown pictures of spiders or snakes, but blank slides, and the shocks were given at pre-arranged times, independently of any physical responses. In other words, the entire procedure was a sham. Nevertheless, the patients in the placebo group showed as much improvement as those undergoing genuine systematic desensitisation. This is not conclusive proof that desensitisation always works entirely by means of the placebo effect, but it does suggest that it has a large placebo component. Perhaps those who claim that modern methods of psychotherapy such as desensitisation and cognitive therapy (which involves teaching patients to identify and overcome negative thought patterns) are much more 'scientific' than earlier methods such as psychoanalysis are not on such firm ground. Just because the theories that the modern methods appeal to are better established does not mean that the methods themselves are less likely to be placebos. A therapy that is based on a true theory of the mind may still turn out to be a placebo, if it does not in fact activate the mechanisms specified in the theory.

THE VALUE OF PSYCHOTHERAPY

From the picture I have painted so far in this chapter, it might seem as if I take an unremittingly dim view of psychotherapy. Surprising as it may seem, that is not true. I do think that the evidence strongly suggests that most, if not all, forms of psychotherapy are pure placebos. I also believe that most of the theories on which the various forms of psychotherapy are based are badly flawed, and in some cases so vacuous as to be 'not even wrong'. And yet, despite all this, I do not think psychotherapy need be an entirely worthless exercise. Sometimes it can be very beneficial. Indeed, I feel that it helped me.

In the early 1990s, when I first became interested in psychoanalysis, I came to the conclusion that I would learn more about the theory if I also experienced something of the practice. So, more out of curiosity than anything else, I found a psychoanalyst and went into treatment. I remember saying in the first session that I could not think of any particular problem I needed help on. Of course I had my fair share of fears and foibles, but none of these amounted to a proper medical *condition*. I wasn't delusional or depressed, nor did I have any of the other classic symptoms of mental disorder. The only complaint I could think of, as I searched in vain for some disease I could offer up as a genuine reason for going to therapy, was a vague sense of writer's block that had been crippling my attempts to write at the time. And guess what? Over the course of the following few months, during which I religiously kept my appointments with my analyst, my writer's block gradually dissolved, and the words began pouring out of me once more.

Of course, the usual caveats apply. I cannot be sure that the psychoanalytic treatment actually caused my writer's block to dissolve; it might have been just a coincidence. But that is not the point of telling this story. Even if we could prove that the treatment was, in fact, the cause of my renewed capacity to write, this would not show that psychoanalysis was any more than a placebo. For writer's block is not really a *disease*. And there is the rub. Psychotherapy may be no better than a placebo at curing diseases, but perhaps that should not be its aim. Critics sometimes sneer that the people who do best out of psychotherapy are those who had nothing wrong with them to begin with. That may well be true – but if so, it does not prove that psychotherapy is useless. It all depends on what you take the aims of psychotherapy to be. If psychotherapy is supposed to be a medical technique, a method for curing mental disorder, then its credentials are not particularly good. But if psychotherapists were to explicitly disavow such pretensions, and promise different benefits instead, their claims might be more accurate.

There are economic reasons, of course, why therapists might not want to take such a radical step. If psychotherapists renounced their claims to be able to cure diseases, the health services that employ them might think twice about renewing their contracts, and those who work privately would probably not attract so many clients. Vague intimations of intangible psychological benefits are much less likely to tempt someone to commit himself to a lengthy and costly course of therapy than concrete promises of better mental health. Yet this is, to my mind at least, the only way that psychotherapists can continue to practise their art and remain honest. And psychotherapists can point to a high degree of consumer satisfaction among their clients. The fact that clients are often very happy with the psychotherapy they receive, even when it has no effect on the original condition for which they first sought help, suggests that clients still value psychotherapy even when it is clear that the benefits are not strictly medical.

Many of those who go to psychotherapy do not have a specific clinical objective in mind, such as relief from panic attacks or overcoming depression. Rather, they want a sympathetic person to listen to their problems. Suggestions that a psychotherapist can do no more than a good friend are sometimes beside the point. For increasingly many people in today's lonely world, a therapist may at times be the only available shoulder to cry on. Even those who are lucky enough to have a good social network of friends and family may prefer a private listening-post to whom secrets can be revealed without fear of the consequences. If this is how psychotherapists described the service they offer, I would have no bone to pick with them at all. Whether or not the state, or medical insurance, should pay for this service is another matter.

We are already beginning to enter the terrain of ethics. All professionals, whether doctors, alternative therapists or psychotherapists, have a duty to describe the services they offer correctly, and clients have a right to be informed. This basic principle seems uncontroversial, yet the existence of the placebo response may suggest that deception is at times legitimate. Indeed, the use of placebos raises a whole range of ethical dilemmas. This is the subject of the next and final chapter.

Chapter 9

THE WITCH DOCTOR'S DILEMMA

Placebos do not just pose scientific problems; they also raise troubling ethical dilemmas. What should alternative therapists and psychotherapists do, for example, if it turns out that they are really purveying placebos? Should they shut up shop and look for some other line of business? Or would it be acceptable for them to carry on with their profession regardless? And what about general practitioners? Is it ethically acceptable for a doctor to give his patients sugar pills and tell them they are potent drugs?

At the heart of all the ethical problems posed by placebos lies a conflict between two moral principles. On the one hand, doctors have a duty to care for their patients and, if possible, cure them of disease. On the other hand, doctors also have a duty to tell their patients the truth. Most of the time, we hope, these two duties are perfectly compatible; but sometimes they pull in different directions.

Even if the placebo effect did not exist, doctors would still face situations in which their duty to care conflicted with their duty to tell the truth. When a patient is found to have an incurable disease, for example, it is not always clear that the doctor should reveal the diagnosis to the patient. Cicero claimed that 'to warn of an evil is justified only if, along with the warning, there is a way of escape'.[1] Perhaps it is better to allow the patient to spend the last few months of his life in blissful ignorance than to burden him with the thought of an impending

181

death when nothing can be done to prevent it. Certainly, there are opposing considerations that will also weigh on the doctor's mind. Warning the patient of his imminent death would at least allow him to put his affairs in order and perhaps do some of the things he has always wanted to do but never got round to doing before. It might even lead him to enjoy the last few months of life more intensely than he would have done otherwise. Still, even if one decides that it is better, on balance, to tell a patient such terrible news, the very fact that this decision is not an easy one points to a potential conflict between the duty to care and the duty to be honest.

The existence of the placebo response makes the dilemma far more acute. For if beliefs can have a direct impact on the functioning of the immune system, then modifying those beliefs by imparting new information to the patient might help or hinder his chance of recovery. If hope itself can cure, and there is little basis for such hope in reality, should the doctor lie to the patient? The medieval French surgeon Henri de Mondeville thought so, and advised doctors to engage in all manner of flowery lies to keep their patients cheerful:

> Keep up your patient's spirits by music of viols and ten-stringed psaltery, or by forged letters describing the death of his enemies, or by telling him that he has been elected to a bishopric, if a churchman.[2]

Few doctors would support the use of such extreme forms of deception today. But often the situation is much more delicately balanced. Many patients do not feel satisfied if they come away from their doctor empty-handed. They do not like to be told that the best way to get better is simply to take it easy for a few days; they want to *do* something about their illness, and a little bottle of pills fits the bill perfectly. In the face of such demands, some doctors may prefer to acquiesce and write out a prescription that they know will have no direct chemical effect on the patient's condition. It is quite tempting, for example, for doctors to prescribe antibiotics for common colds, even though antibiotics are powerless against the viruses that cause such infections. It would surely be better, in such a situation, to prescribe a sugar pill rather than an active drug, especially given the fact that the over-prescription of antibiotics is leading many bacterial infections to develop resistance to them. Neither course of action, however, is completely honest. When it comes to treating common colds, both sugar pills and antibiotics are placebos, and a doctor who gives either to a patient with a runny nose is engaged in an act of deception, albeit a minor one.

PLACEBOS WITHOUT DECEPTION?

The use of placebos does not always involve deceiving the patient. If the doctor is unaware that a particular medicine or technique works only because the patient believes in it, he is not faced with this particular ethical dilemma. He can tell his patients, in all honesty, that the treatment works whether or not they believe in it, because that is what he sincerely believes. Psychotherapy, and many of the various forms of alternative therapy, may be pure placebos, but the therapists who administer them are mostly unaware of this, so they are not guilty of deception. They may, however, be guilty of negligence.

All medical practitioners have a duty to ensure, as far as is practically possible, that their medical knowledge is accurate and up-to-date. The doctors who prescribed thalidomide to pregnant women in the early 1960s could not have known that the drug would lead to serious foetal abnormalities; nobody did. A doctor who prescribed the drug today, however, could not defend himself by claiming that he was unaware of its dangers. For such ignorance would itself be culpable. It takes very little effort to find out about the risks of thalidomide, and a doctor who had not bothered to expend such minimal effort would be seriously negligent.

The law in most countries today does not impose such stringent requirements on psychotherapists and alternative practitioners. Ethically, it seems hard to defend this double standard. Surely psychotherapists and alternative practitioners also have a duty to ensure that their medical knowledge is up-to-date. As should be clear from the two preceding chapters, there is a rapidly accumulating body of scientific evidence which strongly suggests that many forms of psychotherapy and alternative medicine may be pure placebos. It is by no means difficult to access this evidence – a five-minute search on the Internet will suffice to unearth several relevant documents. Psychotherapists and alternative practitioners who are unaware of the various critical studies are burying their heads in the sand. Those who are aware of them, but do not inform their patients of the fact that the treatments they are offering may be pure placebos, are infringing the principle of informed consent.

A SHAMAN'S TRICKS

The ethical dilemmas surrounding the use of placebos are an uncomfortable side-effect of increasing medical knowledge. It is only now that so much information is available about the effects of psychotherapy and alternative medicine that the practitioners who dole out these treatments are faced with difficult choices. Likewise, it was not until Western doctors began to realise, in the nineteenth century, that most of their medicines and therapeutic techniques were at best useless, at worst positively harmful, that they were confronted with a similar dilemma: to renounce the old potions and have nothing to offer the sick and dying – not even hope – or to carry on administering the treatments that they now knew to be inactive.

It is no accident that the surge of interest in placebos after World War II coincided with the advent of modern medicine. By the mid-1940s, the gap between what doctors knew about the causes of disease and their knowledge of efficacious treatments was at its greatest. Useless panaceas such as theriac (whose main ingredient was viper's flesh), and even positively harmful 'remedies' such as bloodletting and leeching, had been the mainstay of medical practice for almost three thousand years before they were gradually abandoned towards the end of the eighteenth century. The founder of scientific pharmacology, Sir John Gaddum, once quipped that *materia medica* was the only field of knowledge that had become smaller as it had advanced.

Still, we must not exaggerate the extent to which doctors were ignorant of the placebo effect before the birth of modern medicine. Long before science provided conclusive proof that many therapeutic techniques could only possibly work – if they did work – by means of the placebo effect, many doctors and healers suspected that this was the case. Witch doctors and shamans, in particular, are far more aware of the role of belief in the cures they perform than they are usually given credit for. After all, the tricks of the trade are transparent to them. They know that the bloody tissue they appear to extract from the patient's body is, in fact, no more than a tuft of down they have been hiding in their own mouth, and the blood is their own, produced by biting their tongue just before they place their lips against the diseased body from which they pretend to suck forth the ailment.

Yet these shamans seem to feel little compunction about engaging in this trickery. The French anthropologist Claude Levi-Strauss tells the story of a shaman called Quesalid, a Kwatiutl Indian from the Vancouver region of Canada.[3] As a young man, Quesalid learned the tricks of the shaman's trade in the traditional way – by being apprenticed to one of the older shamans in his tribe. These practices included the sucking technique just described, as well as a range of other conjuring tricks and fakery, such as simulated fainting and the use of 'dreamers' – that is, spies who listen to private conversations and pass on to the shaman bits of information about the patient, which the shaman then recounts as if he had acquired them by means of some form of extra-sensory perception. When Quesalid is challenged by the shaman of a neighbouring clan to compete with him in attempting to cure several patients, Quesalid emerges triumphant. The other shaman, discredited in the eyes of his fellow clansmen, approaches Quesalid to request an explanation. This shaman is not privy to the secret of the sucking trick, for he uses a different technique in which he simply tells his patients that the illness will pass from their body into his bird-shaped ritual rattle. The trick is a less powerful placebo because it lacks the element of visibility that makes Quesalid's 'bloody worm' so striking. The shaman begs Quesalid to tell him if this, too, is just a trick: 'I pray you to have mercy and tell me what stuck on the palm of your hand last night,' he implores, pitifully. 'Was it the true sickness or was it only made up? For I beg you have mercy and tell me about the way you did it so that I can imitate you.'

The other shaman admits to Quesalid that he does nothing but lie and fake, pretending to practise real magic for the sake of earning a living, stating candidly that he is 'covetous for the property of the sick men'. Quesalid knows that he, too, is a trickster, but he does not let on. That very night, the other shaman leaves his clan, taking his entire family with him, heartsick and ashamed. Quesalid, on the other hand, goes on practising his more elaborate tricks, growing in fame and power, unperturbed by any scruples.

BECOMING MORE OPEN

Shamans and witch doctors guard their secrets carefully, for they know that their tricks would not work if people found out that they were, in fact, just tricks. Western doctors today have a very different ethos, one which values openness and respects the right of the patient to know what the various treatment options are and how they work. The principle of informed consent governs both medical practice and medical research. Patients and participants in clinical trials alike are supposed to be fully informed about the likely risks and benefits of any treatments offered to them, and no treatment should be given unless the recipient freely consents to the procedure. Special rules protect those whose lack of understanding prevents them from giving truly *informed* consent, such as children and the mentally ill, while medical research is forbidden to recruit participants whose consent cannot be regarded as truly free, such as prison inmates.

The principle of informed consent became enshrined in many codes of medical ethics around the world after World War II. Among the various horrors of the Nazi death camps that the Allied forces discovered as they swept across Germany in 1945 were the revelations of medical experiments conducted on the hapless prisoners. In 1947, the trial of twenty-three German physicians and scientists at Nuremberg called witnesses from Nazi hospitals and camps, who recounted details of experiments in which Jews and other prisoners were subjected to freezing temperatures and high altitudes, infected with malaria and typhus, and injected with drugs and poisons – all against their will. This provoked a reaction among the various governing bodies of Western medical associations, who had not previously been so squeamish about matters of informed consent. In the first half of the twentieth century, for example, it was not unknown for medical researchers in the United States to offer prisoners incentives such as free cigarettes to tempt them to take part in experiments on things like the effect of various dietary regimes. While these experiments fell far short of the enforced cruelty of much Nazi research, they were seen by some as the beginning of a slippery slope whose culmination was exemplified by the experiments in the death camps.

The result was a move away from the paternalism that had dominated medicine for centuries – the 'doctor knows best' attitude, rooted in the doctor's monopoly over medical knowledge. In the half-century or so since the end of World War II, doctors have been increasingly encouraged to explain their diagnostic and prescriptive reasoning to their patients, to consult their opinions and listen to their preferences. In 1964, the World Medical Association enshrined the principle of informed consent in the code of ethics that it drew up in Helsinki. This document, which is known as the Declaration of Helsinki, even though it has since been revised at several meetings in other cities, has no legal authority in any country, but still exerts considerable influence over medical authorities around the world. As a result, informed consent has now become a dogma, something that no doctor in his right mind would challenge. Surgeons who operate on patients without first obtaining their consent are struck off, and medical researchers who do not obtain the consent of their subjects do not get their papers published.

Some doctors have argued that Western medicine has become rather too obsessed with the need to inform patients about treatment options. Writing in the *New England Journal of Medicine* in 1980, Franz Ingelfinger argued that 'a certain amount of authoritarianism, paternalism, and domination are the essence of the physician's effectiveness'.[4] Yet surveys show that patients want their physicians to tell them the truth about diagnosis, prognosis and therapy. One survey, for example, found that 90 per cent of patients said they would want to be told of a diagnosis of cancer or Alzheimer's disease.[5] In this age of consumer rights and people power, the old paternalism is no longer appropriate.

Besides, the veil of secrecy that once surrounded medical treatments is rapidly disappearing. Until the late 1990s, doctors were not unlike shamans in the extent to which they had exclusive access to the truth about the tricks of their trade. With the advent of the Internet, however, that has all changed. Nowadays, thousands of websites provide up-to-the-minute information about every condition and treatment, all available at the touch of a button. Anyone with access to a computer can rapidly know more about their ailments than their doctor. Doctors who lie to their patients now run a much higher risk of being caught out.

BEING ECONOMICAL WITH THE TRUTH

In an attempt to reconcile the use of placebos with the ethics of informed consent, some doctors have come up with clever ways of being 'economical with the truth'. Walter Brown, a professor of psychiatry at Brown University, suggests that doctors prescribing placebos could say something along the lines of the following: 'Mrs Jones, the type of depression you have has been treated in the past with either antidepressant medicine or psychotherapy, one of the talking therapies. These two treatments are still widely used and are options for you. There is a third kind of treatment, less expensive for you and less likely to cause side-effects, which also helps many people with your condition. This treatment involves taking one of these pills twice a day and coming to our office every two weeks to let us know how you're doing. These pills do not contain any drug. We don't know exactly how they work; they may trigger or stimulate the body's own healing processes. We do know that your chances of improving with this treatment are quite good. If after six weeks of this treatment you're not feeling better we can try one of the other treatments.'[6]

Brown claims that this script satisfies the principle of informed consent, while simultaneously preserving the belief that is a vital prerequisite for the placebo effect to take place. To others, the form of words Brown has crafted still smacks of dishonesty. Perhaps, however, there is no need for any trickery at all. In one study conducted in 1965, two researchers from Johns Hopkins University gave placebos to fifteen patients with neurotic disorders without even attempting to conceal the truth.[7] 'We feel that a so-called sugar pill may help you,' they told their patients. 'Do you know what a sugar pill is? A sugar pill is a pill with no medicine at all in it. I think this pill will help you as it has helped so many others. Are you willing to try this pill?' Fourteen of the patients agreed to take the sugar pills (the fifteenth refused after her husband laughed at the idea), and thirteen improved during the week of taking them. As a no-treatment group was not included in the study, we cannot be sure if this improvement was due in part to the placebo effect, or whether it was due entirely to spontaneous remission and the natural course of the disease. However, the fact that several patients, including one who had been suicidal, improved a great deal, suggests that the placebo effect played some part. So perhaps deception is not necessary at all.

The fact that placebos can work even if patients know what they are being given is hard to explain. One possibility is that patients do not, in fact, believe what the doctor tells them. When the patients involved in the study just cited were questioned, some said that they were sure the doctors had been lying to them. Nobody, they argued, would be daft enough to prescribe mere sugar pills to anxious patients; the psychiatrists must, they thought, be secretly testing powerful drugs on them.

This story nicely illustrates the complexities of putting the principle of informed consent into practice. Simply telling patients that they will be given a placebo may not be enough: they may doubt the doctor's word, or misunderstand the term placebo. Calling it a sugar pill is probably less likely to mislead, but even here patients may not be aware of all the risks. They may not realise, for example, the value of the treatments they are forgoing by choosing to take a placebo instead of, say, a proven antidepressant. Patients may be much better informed today than they were even a decade ago, but this does not mean they are always in full possession of all the relevant facts. Insisting on informed consent may be necessary to preserve the patient's rights, but it is not sufficient by itself to guarantee those rights.

WHEN PLACEBOS ARE NOT JUSTIFIED

The moral dilemmas posed by placebos depend for their bite on the power and extent of the placebo response. If it is as powerful and ubiquitous as some have claimed, this might well tip the scales in favour of the duty to care for the patient, at the expense of the doctor's duty to tell the truth – if not always, then at least on some occasions. If, however, I am right in claiming that the placebo response only affects a handful of conditions – pain, swelling, depression and other manifestations of the acute phase response – then the ethical dilemma loses much of its force. When treating any other medical condition apart from those that are placebo-responsive, the case for knowingly prescribing a placebo is much less convincing. In these cases, prescribing a placebo would bring no benefit to the patient's health, and consequently it would be hard to see how a doctor could justify lying to his patient without such a benefit. Cancer, for example, is almost certainly not placebo-responsive. There can be no justification, therefore, in handing out placebos to those suffering from any of the various forms of this particular disease.

Even when a condition is known to be placebo-responsive, however, there are reasons to doubt that the benefit provided to the patient by a placebo is great enough to justify prescribing one. As Austin Bradford Hill, one of the pioneers of clinical trials, pointed out in 1963, the ethical status of prescribing placebos depends in large part on the alternative treatments available to the doctor.[8] Before World War II, when there were so few effective drugs in existence, which only worked for a handful of medical conditions, it was perhaps more justifiable to engage in the 'pious fraud' of handing out bread pills and inactive 'tonics'. When the choice was simply between no treatment at all, and a placebo that was at worst harmless and might, possibly, do some good, doctors who chose the latter option were making the best of a bad situation.

The situation is very different today. When so many treatments of proven value exist for a whole range of medical conditions, it seems inherently wrong to prescribe a placebo instead. A depressed patient may get some relief from a placebo, but if he takes Prozac he will get more. This is yet another consideration that raises serious ethical doubts about the continuing practice of psychotherapy and alternative medicine. A patient who visits a psychotherapist or a homeopath may feel that this removes the need to visit an orthodox doctor. Even if he has a placebo-responsive condition, and the therapy does him some good, a less effective treatment has been substituted for a more effective one.

THE USE OF PLACEBOS IN CLINICAL TRIALS

One ethical principle governing the use of placebos, then, is that they should not be used when a superior treatment is readily available. This principle is rarely flouted by orthodox practitioners, except in the context of medical research. When a new treatment is developed for a condition that is already treatable by a proven drug, the patients in the trial are effectively deprived of a proven remedy.[9] In 1985, for example, a group of investigators conducted a trial of a drug called ivermectin for river blindness. The drug was tested against a placebo even though another drug of known efficacy – diethylcarbamazine – was readily available. The participants in the trial were illiterate Liberian seamen, some of whom indicated their 'informed consent' by thumbprint.[10] Dozens of other trials concerning drugs for all sorts of conditions also continue to use placebo control groups even though a proven therapy already exists.

This practice was condemned by the Declaration of Helsinki until October 2000, when the World Medical Association drafted an amendment calling for new drugs to be tested against 'the best current treatment'. According to the revised document, known as the Edinburgh revision, a new drug should be tested against a placebo only when no proven treatment is currently available. Perhaps unsurprisingly, the amendment was not greeted with great delight by the pharmaceutical companies. It is, after all, easier to prove that a new drug is superior to a placebo than to prove that it is superior to the best current treatment. In July 2000, just a few months before the Helsinki Declaration was amended, the International Conference on Harmonisation of Technical Requirements for Registration of Pharmaceuticals for Human Use released a document explicitly stating that placebo use is generally acceptable in clinical trials. Clearly, there is room for a lot of disagreement.

The Edinburgh revision of the Declaration of Helsinki has problems of its own.[11] It ruled out placebo-controlled trials for conditions in which a proven treatment was currently available, on the grounds that such trials would deprive all the participants of an effective remedy. Neither those in the placebo arm, nor those in the experimental arm, would be given the standard medical treatment available to patients not involved in the trial. But the recommendation instead of trials with 'active control groups' is only half a solution. In such trials, the control group does not receive a placebo but instead is given the standard treatment – which has, presumably, already been shown to be superior to a placebo. But the patients in the experimental group *are* still deprived of the standard treatment. They are offered an as-yet unproven treatment instead of a therapy that has already been shown to work. The Edinburgh revision, then, continues to approve of trials in which some participants, at least, are deprived of the best current treatment.

Those who defend the use of placebos in clinical trials, even when a treatment of proven value already exists, usually appeal to the principle of informed consent. So long as patients are fully informed about the risks of entering a trial, and still agree to participate, the argument goes, there is no reason to prevent them from doing so. Critics object that patients rarely – if ever – understand their treatment options and the trial design well enough to be able to make fully informed decisions. Nor does this consideration just apply to extreme cases, such as the trial referred to earlier involving the Liberian fishermen. Even when careful measures are taken to inform patients of the risks involved in clinical trials, it is doubtful that patients really know what they are getting into. The consent forms handed out to potential participants in clinical trials are complex affairs, designed more to shield the investigators from possible lawsuits than to provide a balanced overview of the risks of entering the trial. It seems hard to avoid the conclusion that placebo control groups are unethical unless placebos are thought to be the best current treatment for the condition in question.

There is one way of using placebos in clinical trials that does not flout this principle. Some clinical trials, known as 'add-on' trials, give all participants the standard treatment as a baseline. In addition to this, half of the participants receive the experimental treatment, while the others receive a placebo. The use of placebos in add-on trials is much more ethically acceptable because nobody is deprived of the best current therapy. Everyone gets it, and the placebo is only used to ensure proper double-blinding.

SHAM SURGERY

If giving patients dummy pills is morally dubious, then giving them sham surgery may seem an outright offence. The official policy of the US Food and Drug Administration reflects this view: placebo-controlled trials are usually required before new drugs can be approved, but new surgical techniques are not so tightly supervised.

One reason for this double standard is practical. It is much harder to ensure uniformity in surgical procedures than in drug treatment, and trials are therefore harder to standardise. Each operation is different, because the details of each patient's body are different. All surgery has an element of experimentation, and it is hard to say at which point official scrutiny should begin. Far more pressing than these practical considerations are the moral ones. The ethical dilemmas raised by the use of placebos in clinical trials become even more perplexing when you move away from drug trials and consider instead trials of surgical procedures. Those who receive placebos in drug trials may suffer by omission – they are deprived of the possible benefit of the experimental treatment, for example – but the placebo itself will not do them any direct harm. In trials of surgical procedures, however, patients who receive the dummy operation are exposed to all the usual dangers of surgery – the risk of infection, postoperative pain and so on – for no tangible benefit. This has led many medical researchers to assume that placebo-controlled trials of surgical procedures are beyond the pale.

Some researchers are beginning to question this received wisdom. With the advent of less invasive surgical techniques, the risk of infection and the severity of postoperative pain are now much lower, making the cost–benefit analysis of sham surgery more evenly balanced. And the benefits, say the proponents of surgical trials, are not negligible. If a trial shows that a surgical procedure is no better than a placebo, it can be removed from medical practice, thus sparing thousands of future patients unnecessary operations. Recall the example of internal mammary ligation, which we looked at briefly in Chapter Two. In the 1940s and 1950s, thousands of patients underwent this painful procedure, which involved cutting into the chest and tying knots in some of the arteries supplying blood to the heart. It certainly seemed to work: three-quarters of all patients who underwent the operation improved. Then, in the late 1950s, two pioneering studies tried a sham version of the operation, which involved cutting into the chest but not tying knots in any arteries, and found that the results of this dummy procedure were just as impressive. This led doctors to abandon the operation, thereby saving thousands more patients from unnecessary surgery.

In a more recent example, a surgeon at the Baylor College of Medicine in Houston, Texas, carried out a small placebo-controlled trial of arthroscopy.[12] This operation, which involves scraping and rinsing the knee joint, is carried out on patients with arthritis in their knees. It generally works, leading to prolonged pain relief, but J. Bruce Moseley wanted to find out *why* it worked. Did the procedure, he wondered, work entirely by means of the placebo effect? Moseley took ten volunteers – all former military men – but only gave the standard operation to two of them. Three received only the rinsing, without the scraping, and five received only a small incision, with no rinsing *or* scraping. Nobody knew who would get the real operation and who would get the placebo until the volunteers were in the operating theatre and Moseley opened an envelope with secret instructions. Since the volunteers were fully anaesthetised by that point, and Moseley didn't tell them afterwards what he had done, the patients remained unaware whether they had received the real operation or the sham. Six months later, they still couldn't guess. All reported a significant decrease in pain, and all were happy with their operations. This was only a pilot study – the small number of patients makes it impossible to say for sure that there is really no difference between arthroscopy and placebo – but it was enough to convince Moseley to set up a much bigger study that could provide more definitive conclusions.

Moseley justifies his experiment with the same reasoning that was used to legitimise the trials of internal mammary ligation in the 1950s. The scraping and rinsing of the knee joint involved in arthroscopic knee surgery usually requires general anaesthesia, which is still a rather risky procedure. If, however, the same amount of pain relief could be produced with a mere incision, which can be performed with a mere sedative, then future patients could be spared the risks of general anaesthesia. The problem with this type of moral calculation is that it weighs a benefit for future patients against a cost for present patients. Yet this may be an inevitable feature of all medical research. As the World Medical Association stated in the Declaration of Helsinki, 'medical progress is based on research which ultimately must rest in part on experimentation involving human subjects'.

PROTECTING THE PUBLIC

Placebos do not just create private moral dilemmas for doctors and medical researchers; they also raise ethical questions for society as a whole. If I am right in my analysis of alternative medicine and psychotherapy, there are hundreds of thousands of people purveying placebos in the Western world, let alone in the developing countries. To what extent, and how, should governments try to protect their citizens from quackery?

THE WITCH DOCTOR'S DILEMMA

During the 1970s many governments in the West brought into effect legislation that required all new drugs to be tested in clinical trials before doctors could use them. This new regulatory regime was designed to protect the public, but it is easy to see that it is only a half-measure. For one thing, it imposed a much higher burden of proof on pharmacotherapy than on other kinds of treatment for which controlled trials are difficult or unethical to run. It is hard, as we have seen, to construct adequate controls for most forms of psychotherapy, and there are ethical problems with introducing placebo controls in clinical trials of surgical procedures. As a result, there is a double standard in the evaluation of therapeutic resources. On the one hand, drugs are not allowed to be used unless they pass extremely stringent clinical trials. On the other, many surgical procedures and most forms of psychotherapy are permitted despite scant efforts to explore their efficacy.

There has been, as we have seen, an increase in serious research into the effects of psychotherapy and alternative medicine, but the results of that research are at best ambiguous. If a new drug received such scant empirical support during initial clinical trials, it is doubtful that it would be granted a licence. Yet psychotherapy and alternative medicine are unregulated in many countries, and where regulation does exist, it is not very stringent. It is hard to see how this situation can be justified.

It could be argued that imposing tighter controls on psychotherapy and alternative medicine would infringe people's rights to treat themselves in the way they wish. If people want to spend their money on unproven remedies, what right do governments have to stop them? The libertarian can always argue that those who visit alternative practitioners *choose* to do so, and, while we can always argue with such choices, we have an ethical duty to respect them. However, it is doubtful that such choices are always truly free, because they are often made by people who are not in full possession of the relevant facts. Those who consult psychotherapists and practitioners of alternative medicine are not usually aware of the empirical evidence concerning those treatments' effectiveness. If orthodox doctors are not always as scrupulous as they should be about obtaining informed consent, they are at least far ahead of psychotherapists and alternative practitioners, who typically give very little accurate information to their patients about the chances of successful treatment, the range of other treatments available (including orthodox ones), and the risks of using one approach rather than another. It seems unfair, to say the least, to focus all our criticism on orthodox medicine, when alternative practitioners are guilty of even greater infringements of the patient's right to know.

When statutory health warnings are attached to cigarette packets, should they not also be compulsory for all those forms of alternative medicine that are so widely available today? Perhaps homeopathic remedies should be sold with a label reading: 'Warning: this product is a placebo. It will work only if you believe in homeopathy, and only for certain conditions such as pain and depression. Even then, it is not likely to be as powerful as orthodox drugs. You may get fewer side-effects from this treatment than from a drug, but you will probably also get less benefit.'

Fans of alternative medicine might baulk at such a suggestion, but that would smack of prejudice. As medical decision-making becomes an increasingly co-operative venture involving patients as equal partners in the prescription process, providing them with accurate information about the various remedies available becomes of the utmost importance. This applies just as much to alternative medicine and psychotherapy as it does to the various resources of orthodox medicine.

CONCLUSION

During the 1980s, a biochemist called Wilson Harvey was working on the cellular effects of therapeutic ultrasound — commonly used for treating a variety of soft-tissue injuries. Part of this research was to check that the ultrasound machines were functional and emitting the correct intensity of sound. It was a task that hardly seemed necessary, as both staff and patients reported that the machines gave great benefit. When Harvey checked the machines, however, he found that some of them were emitting levels of ultrasound far below the prescribed amount. One was not emitting any ultrasound at all.

It was this discovery that led Harvey and his colleagues, some years later, to conduct the experiments comparing real and 'fake' ultrasound which we looked at briefly in Chapter Two. To recap briefly, in one experiment Harvey and colleagues took 150 patients who had undergone dental surgery, and divided them into several groups.[1] Some received the real ultrasound treatment. Others were massaged with the ultrasound machine while it was turned off, while another group received no treatment at all. Curiously, postoperative pain and swelling were reduced in all patients treated with the ultrasound machine — whether it was turned on or off. Harvey and his colleagues concluded that much, if not all of the effect of ultrasound treatment was due to the placebo effect. The reason ultrasound worked was simply because the patients *believed* it worked.

During their coffee breaks, Harvey and his colleagues would

sometimes amuse themselves with an instructive thought-experiment. What, they asked, would be the ingredients of the ideal placebo? Various suggestions were mooted. Some felt that lots of impressive technology and gadgetry was important. This seemed to be crucial not only in explaining the success of ultrasound treatment – with its gleaming white machinery – but also perhaps played a part in other high-tech means of pain relief such as TENS (transcutaneous electrical nerve stimulation). Others argued instead that the most important ingredient was the physician, and that his power to evoke the placebo response would be augmented by cloaking him in the paraphernalia of medical authority. Others agreed that the physician was indeed the most important element, but felt that his power to elicit the placebo response lay more in his capacity to demonstrate concern and sympathy – perhaps by his reassuring tone of voice, or by spending more time with the patient, or by direct physical contact. Perhaps, indeed, the act of touching and manipulating the patient was itself a powerful ingredient in the placebo response, irrespective of how this was interpreted by the patient.

All these suggestions are plausible, but they are all subject to an important qualification. Technology, medical authority and even sympathy can only play their part in helping to elicit the placebo response *indirectly*, by virtue of the effect they have on the patient's *beliefs*. Placebos only work to the extent that patients believe they work, so anything that enhances the credibility of a particular kind of treatment will boost the capacity of that treatment to evoke the placebo response. Ultimately, it is the *belief* in the treatment that sets off the placebo response. And belief is something that lies inside the patient's mind. All the other 'ingredients' of the ideal placebo – the external trappings, such as technology and the paraphernalia of medical authority – only work by increasing the patient's belief in the efficacy of the treatment.

This explains why the thought-experiment that Harvey and his colleagues used to amuse themselves with could never have led to a consensus. For belief is a subjective affair, varying greatly from person to person. The very factors that may *enhance* the credibility of a particular treatment in *my* eyes may *detract* from its credibility in *yours*. To a firm believer in the power of Western medicine, a gleaming white machine with lots of buttons may be the essence of a powerful treatment. To a committed practitioner of alternative medicine, however, or to a member of a remote indigenous tribe, other kinds of apparatus may be much more credible. Likewise, the paraphernalia that symbolise medical authority differ from culture to culture: a white coat may work in America or Britain, but in some parts of Africa or Asia a great healer would wear a very different kind of apparel.

The ideal placebo, therefore, will differ from person to person. What works for me may not work for you. This is almost certainly one reason why there has been so much variability in studies of the placebo effect. Another reason, as has been seen, is that not all medical conditions are placebo-responsive. But even if we restrict ourselves to studies of conditions such as pain, swelling and depression, which do seem to respond to placebos, there is still a great deal of variability in the extent of the placebo response. How could it be otherwise, when there are so many factors that potentially affect the credibility of any particular medical treatment?

According to one popular view, science proceeds by reducing variability to regularity. It uncovers the sources of variation one by one, and proposes laws that allow us to predict, on the basis of these sources, what the final outcome will be. If so, we must admit that we are still far from achieving a scientific understanding of the placebo response. Too many unknown factors are involved to allow us to make anything more than a vague guess about how powerful a particular placebo will be for a particular patient.

Nevertheless, some progress has been made. As we saw in Chapter Four, various experiments have manipulated the kinds of evidence people are exposed to, in order to influence, in turn, their degree of belief in the efficacy of a particular kind of treatment. To recall just one such experiment, Nicholas Voudouris, a psychologist at La Trobe University in Australia, tricked volunteers into believing that a simple cold cream had potent analgesic effects by presenting them with false evidence about its efficacy.[2] The volunteers underwent a series of pain-tolerance tests with the cream applied, and for each test the length of time they could withstand the pain was measured. Unknown to the volunteers, however, the machine used to induce the pain was turned down whenever the cream was applied, so it appeared to them as if the cream was really blocking the pain. Finally, the volunteers were given two more tests – one with the cream applied, and one without – during which the machine was turned back up. Sure enough, the volunteers were able to tolerate the pain much longer when the cream was applied in the final test than when it had been applied in the initial test. They had learned from the apparently incontrovertible testimony of their own experience that the cream was a powerful painkiller, and this newly acquired belief triggered the placebo response.

If we are to understand the ways in which people come to believe in the power of medicine, experiments like this are vital. But forming a belief in the potency of a particular treatment is only the first step in the chain of events that constitute a full-fledged placebo response. Once the belief has been formed, it must somehow activate the complex series of biochemical pathways involved in suppressing the acute phase response. This step, too, needs to be understood in much more detail before we can claim to have a good scientific understanding of how placebos work. As immunologists and neuroscientists collaborate in teasing apart the various molecular messengers that allow the brain to communicate with the immune system, these details are gradually beginning to emerge. But there is still a long way to go, and the details are fiendishly complicated.

In addition to studying the sources of belief in medicine, and the mechanisms that translate this belief into precise physiological effects, understanding the placebo response also requires knowing how these physiological effects impact on the course of various medical conditions. Here, with this third and final part of the puzzle of the placebo response, there may be some greater hope for regularity – if, that is, the hypothesis proposed in this book turns out to be true. I have argued that placebos work by suppressing the acute phase response, and therefore that they will only help alleviate those medical conditions that involve the activation of the acute phase response. This hypothesis at least has the merit of being fairly lawlike. Yet, as we have seen at several points, the relationship between the acute phase response and various medical conditions is itself a complex thing. Depression, for example, may not seem at first sight to involve the acute phase response, but Michael Maes and his colleagues have published evidence that the same chemical messenger that plays a starring role in exporting local inflammation to the brain and triggering the psychological symptoms of the acute phase response after infection – IL-1ß – is also produced in greater amounts by macrophages in the blood of severely depressed people.[3] This evidence is still far from conclusive, and Maes' conclusions are not universally accepted among immunologists, but it does at least provide some grounds for thinking that the acute phase response is involved in a wider range of medical conditions than has previously been thought. If it turns out that the range of medical conditions involving activation of the acute phase response coincides with the range of conditions that respond to placebos, another important part of the jigsaw puzzle will fall into place.

The daunting complexity of the picture that is emerging from scientific research into the placebo response presents a strong contrast with the simplistic messages touted by many of those in the alternative health movement. The power of the mind to heal the body is regularly affirmed, as if the mind could cure any and every affliction, without regard to the ambiguities and caveats of hard scientific evidence. 'You can heal your life!' proclaims the New Age guru Louise Hay, who claims that she cured herself of cancer simply by changing her own thought patterns.[4]

There is, of course, great comfort to be had from the idea that the mind's power to heal the body is unlimited. Truth and comfort, however, do not always make good bedfellows. And the best guide to truth in these matters is painstaking scientific research, not the wild pronouncements of prophets and gurus. Unfortunately, the scientific evidence does not back up the claims of Louise Hay and other fervent believers in the power of the mind. Cancer is a case in point. By the time they have grown large enough to be detected, most tumours are probably too well established to be eliminated by the body's natural killer cells. So even if these cells turn out to be as responsive to psychological input as some immunologists now claim, this would not mean that the mind could cure an established cancer.

Still, all is not doom and gloom. The falsity of the grand claims made by Hay and others should not lead us to ignore the less dramatic, but still impressive, findings of recent scientific research in mind-body medicine. The power of the mind to heal the body may not be unlimited, but nor is it negligible. As we have seen, some medical conditions are susceptible to a direct effect of the mind on the immune system, as when a placebo causes a belief to emerge which then suppresses the acute phase response. And even if some diseases, such as cancer, are not susceptible to such a direct effect, a positive mental attitude can still attack them indirectly, by making patients more likely to take all the available steps to fight their disease. The mind fights disease in many ways, and the most important of these is still by prompting us to take the right *action*.

NOTES

PREFACE
1 Anonymous, 1973: 35
2 Blalock, 1984

1: PLACEBOS ON TRIAL
1 Healey, 1997: 89
2 Wolff et al., 1946
3 Lasagna, 1955
4 Anonymous, 1954
5 Beecher, 1955
6 Kienle and Kiene, 1997
7 Greenhalgh, 2001: ix
8 Lilienfeld, 1982: 4
9 Kruger et al., 1987
10 Healey, 1997: 90
11 Ibid.: 100
12 Sackett et al., 1996
13 Buckman and Sabbagh, 1993: 246
14 Martin, 1997: 250
15 Ernst, 1994: 33
16 Ernst and Resch, 1995
17 Kienle and Kiene, 1997
18 Spiegel et al., 1989
19 Spiegel, 1997
20 Klopfer, 1957
21 Weil, 1995: 47
22 Cited in Burne, 2000: 15
23 Greenhalgh, 2001: 54
24 Shapiro, 1994: 771

2: WHAT CAN PLACEBOS REALLY DO?
1 Buckman and Sabbagh, 1993: 246
2 Shapiro and Shapiro, 1997: 27
3 Kienle and Kiene, 1997
4 Hrobjartsson and Gotzsche, 2001
5 Spiro, 1997: 37
6 Hashish et al., 1986
7 Ibid.
8 Benedetti et al., 1998
9 Branthwaite and Cooper, 1981
10 Diamond et al, 1958; Cobb et al., 1959
11 Buckman and Sabbagh, 1993: 186–7
12 Abbot, 1952
13 Hashish et. al., 1986; Hashish et al., 1988
14 Moerman, 2000
15 de Craen et al., 1999
16 Schapira, et al., 1970
17 Kirsch and Sapirstein, 1998
18 Klein, 1998
19 Rabkin et al., 1986
20 Fisher and Greenberg, 1993
21 Ibid.
22 Lehmann, 1993

3: THE ACUTE PHASE RESPONSE
1 Kent et al., 1992
2 Baumann and Gauldie, 1994
3 Wall, 1999b: 52
4 Baumann and Gauldie, 1994
5 Bartfai, 2001
6 Maier and Watkins, 1998: 86
7 Kluger et al., 2001: 690–1
8 Kluger, 1979
9 Charlton, 2000
10 Maes et al., 1991
11 Evans et al., 2000: 88–9
12 Maier et al., 2001: 577
13 Levine et al., 1978
14 Wall, 1999a: 1419
15 Alem, 1987
16 Brown, 2001
17 Lynn, 1988
18 Buckman and Sabbagh, 1993: 178–179
19 Motluk, 1999
20 Ibid.

4: THE BELIEF EFFECT
1 Fuente-Fernandez et al., 2001
2 Cherniak, 1986: 6
3 Russell, 1971: 311
4 Martin, 1997: 100
5 Wickramasekera, 1980
6 Voudouris et al., 1989
7 Montgomery and Kirsch, 1997
8 Beecher, 1955
9 McQuay et al., 1995
10 Kirschbaum et al., 1992
11 Gracely et al., 1985
12 Hay, 1984: 221
13 Ibid.: 2

5: WHY? THE EVOLUTIONARY QUESTION
1 Nesse and Williams, 1994
2 Ibid.: 123–4
3 Morgan, 1990
4 Ader and Cohen, 1975

5 Ibid.
6 Bovbjerg et al., 1990
7 Herrnstein, 1962
8 Longo et al., 1999
9 Smith and McDaniels, 1983
10 Blalock, 1984
11 Porter, 1997: 44–50
12 Ibid.: 35
13 Wall, 1999b: 155
14 Humphrey, 2000

6: NOCEBO – BEYOND GOOD AND BAD
1 Buckman and Sabbagh, 1993: 246
2 Ibid.: 125–6
3 Beecher, 1955: 1603
4 Blackwell et al., 1972
5 Rosenzweig et al., 1993
6 Kennedy, 1961
7 Cannon, 1942
8 Wall, 1999b: 114
9 Taylor, 1996: 65–6
10 Oswald Savage, cited in Le Fanu, 1999: 23
11 Haggard, 1934, 267–8, cited in Shapiro and Shapiro, 1997b: 22
12 Schmitt, 1980
13 Crocetti et al., 2001
14 Pütsep et al., 1999
15 Hamilton, 2001
16 Nesse, 2000: 16
17 Wolpert and Evans, 2001
18 Sapolsky et al., 1997
19 Maier and Watkins, 1998

7: THE ALTERNATIVES
1 Ernst, 1996
2 Burne, 2000
3 Survey by ICM research for BBC Radio 5 Live, August 1999
4 Watkins and Lewith, 1997
5 BMA Board of Science and Education, 2000

6 Burne, 2000
7 House of Lords Select
   Committee on Science and
   Technology, 2000
8 BMA Board of Science and
   Education, 2000
9 Patel, 1987
10 Launso, 1994
11 Vickers, 1996
12 Diamond, 2001: 58–60
13 Linde et al., 1997
14 Bobak and Donald, 1998
15 Gratzer, 2000
16 Samal and Geckeler, 2001
17 Davenas et al., 1988; see also
   Endler and Schulte, 1994
18 Benveniste, 1998
19 Maddox et al., 1988
20 Galloway, 2001: 561
21 Vickers, 1996: 14
22 Dale and Cornwell, 1994
23 Kaptchuk et al, 1996
24 Talbot, 2000
25 Davies, 1996
26 Randi, 1989

8: PSYCHOTHERAPY – THE
PUREST PLACEBO?
1 Eysenck, 1952
2 American Handbook of Psychiatry,
   cited in Dineen, 1999: 97
3 Smith and Glass, 1977
4 Smith et al., 1980
5 Prioleau et al., 1983
6 Strupp and Hadley, 1979

7 Stein and Lambert, 1984
8 Smith et al., 1980
9 Epstein, 1985: 130, n.1
10 Kleinman, 1988: 112
11 Cited in Talbot, 2000
12 Glover, 1955: vii
13 DeMarco, 1988: 211
14 Lick, 1975

9: THE WITCH DOCTOR'S
DILEMMA
1 Cicero, 1964: 433 (De
   Divinatione Book II, sec.XXV)
2 Cited in Garrison, 1929: 156
3 Levi-Strauss, 1968: 175–178
4 Ingelfinger, 1980
5 Ethics in medicine: University
   of Washington School of
   Medicine website: http://
   eduserv.hscer.washington.edu/
   bioethics/topics/truth. html
6 Talbot, 2000
7 Park and Covi, 1965
8 Hill, 1963
9 Senn, 2001
10 Greene et al., 1985
11 Senn, 2001
12 Moseley et al., 1996

CONCLUSION
1 Hashish et al., 1986
2 Voudouris et al., 1989
3 Maes et al., 1991
4 Hay, 1984

BIBLIOGRAPHY

Abbot, F.K., M. Mack et al. (1952). The action of banthine on the stomach and duodenum of man with observations on the effects of placebos. *Gastroenterology* 20: 249–261

Ader, R. and N. Cohen (1975). Behaviorally conditioned immunosuppression. *Psychosomatic Medicine* 37: 333–340

Alem, M.A.A.A. (1987). Placebo mechanisms in the treatment of post-operative morbidity. MSc Thesis, Eastman Dental Hospital, University College London

Anonymous (1954). The humble humbug. *Lancet* ii: 321

Anonymous (1973). *The Dhammapada.* Harmondsworth, Penguin

Bartfai, T. (2001). Telling the brain about pain. *Nature* 410: 425–427

Baumann, H. and J. Gauldie (1994). The acute phase response. *Immunology Today* 15(2): 74–80

Beecher, H.K. (1955). The powerful placebo. *Journal of the American Medical Association* 159: 1602–6

Benedetti, F., M. Amanzio et al. (1998). The specific effects of prior opioid exposure on placebo analgesia and placebo respiratory depression. *Pain* 75: 313–319

Benveniste, J. (1998). Meta-analysis of homeopathy trials (correspondence). *Lancet* 351

Berman, J.S. and N.C. Norton (1985). Does professional training make a therapist more effective? *Psychological Bulletin* 98: 401–407

Blackwell, B., S.S. Bloomfield et al. (1972). Demonstration to medical students of placebo responses and non-drug factors. *Lancet* 1: 1279–1282

Blalock, J.E. (1984). The immune system as a sensory organ. *Journal of Immunology* 132(3): 1067–1070

BMA Board of Science and Education (2000). *Acupuncture: Efficacy, Safety and Practice.* London, Harwood

Bobak, M. and A. Donald (1998). Meta-analysis of homeopathy trials (correspondence). *Lancet* 351

Bovbjerg, D.H., W.H. Redd et al. (1990). Anticipatory immune suppression and nausea in women receiving cyclic chemotherapy for ovarian cancer. *Journal of Consulting and Clinical Psychology* 58: 153–157

Branthwaite, A. and P. Cooper (1981). Analgesic effects of branding in treatment of headaches. *British Medical Journal* 282: 1576–1578

Brown, P. (2001). Cinderella goes to the ball. *Nature* 410: 1018–1020

Buckman, R. and K. Sabbagh (1993). *Magic or Medicine? An Investigation of Healing and Healers.* London, Pan Books

Burne, J. (2000). Healing in Harmony. *Guardian* 26 February 2000, Weekend section, 9–17

Cannon, W.B. (1942). Voodoo death. *American Anthropologist* 44(2): 169–181

Charlton, B.G. (2000). The malaise theory of depression: major depressive disorder is sickness behavior and antidepressants are analgesic. *Medical Hypotheses* 54: 1–5

Cherniak, C. (1986). *Minimal Rationality.* Cambridge, MA and London, MIT Press

Cicero (1964). *De Divinatione.* Cambridge, MA, Harvard University Press

Cobb, L.A., G.I. Thomas et al. (1959). An evaluation of internal mammary artery ligation by a double-blind technic. *New England Journal of Medicine* 20: 1115–1118

Crocetti, M., N. Moghbeli et al. (2001). Fever phobia revisited: have parental misconceptions about fever changed in 20 years? *Pediatrics* 107(6): 1241–1246

Dale, A. and S. Cornwell (1994). The role of lavender oil in relieving perineal discomfort following childbirth: a blind, randomised clinical trial. *Journal of Advanced Nursing* 19: 89–96

Davenas, E., F. Beauvais et al. (1988). Human basophil degranulation triggered by very dilute antiserum against IgE. *Nature* 333: 816–818

Davies, R. (1996). *The Merry Heart.* Toronto, McClelland & Stewart

de Craen, A.J., D.E. Moerman et al. (1999). Placebo effect in the treatment of duodenal ulcer. *British Journal of Clinical Pharmacology* 48: 853–60

DeMarco, C.W. (1988). On the impossibility of placebo effects in psychotherapy. *Philosophical Psychology* 11(2): 207–227

Diamond, E.G., C.F. Kittle et al. (1958). Evaluation of internal mammary ligation and sham procedure in angina pectoris. *Circulation* 18: 712–713

Diamond, J. (2001). *Snake Oil.* London, Vintage

Dineen, T. (1999). *Manufacturing Victims: What the Psychology Industry is Doing to People.* London, Constable

Dormandy, T.L. (1988). In praise of peroxidation. *Lancet* 2: 1126–8

Dubinsky, M. and J.H. Ferguson (1990). Analysis of the National Institutes of Health Medicare coverage assessment. *International Journal of Technology and Assessment in Health Care* 6: 480–8

Endler, P.C. and J. Schulte (1994). *Ultra-High Dilution: Physiology and Physics*. Dordrecht, Kluwer

Epstein, W.M. (1985). *The Illusion of Psychotherapy*. New Brunswick, Transaction

Ernst, E. (1994). Placebo: what would we do without it? *European Journal of Physical Medicine and Rehabilitation* 4: 33

Ernst, E. (1996). Direct risks associated with complementary therapies. *Complementary Medicine: An Objective Appraisal*. Ed. E. Ernst. Oxford, Butterworth-Heinemann: 112–125

Ernst, E. and K.L. Resch (1995). Concept of true and perceived placebo effects. *British Medical Journal* 311: 551–3

Evans, P., F. Hucklebridge et al. (2000). *Mind, Immunity and Health: The Science of Psychoneuroimmunology*. London and New York, Free Association Books

Eysenck, H.J. (1952). The effects of psychotherapy: an evaluation. *Journal of Consulting Psychology* 16: 319–24

Fisher, S. and R.P. Greenberg (1993). How sound is the double-blind design for evaluating psychotropic drugs? *Journal of Nervous and Mental Disease* 181(6): 345–350

Fuente-Fernandez, R. de la., T.J. Ruth et al. (2001). Expectation and dopamine release: mechanism of the placebo effect in Parkinson's disease. *Science* 293: 1164–1166

Galloway, J. (2001). Getting the point across. *Nature* 409: 560–1

Garrison, F.H. (1929). *An Introduction to the History of Medicine* (4th edition). Philadelphia, W.B. Saunders

Glover, E. (1955). *The Technique of Psychoanalysis*. New York, International Universities Press

Gracely, R.H., R. Dubner et al. (1985). Clinicians' expectations influence placebo analgesia. *Lancet* 1: 43

Gratzer, W. (2000). The biotechnologist's jungle book. *Nature* 406: 235–236

Greene, B.M., H.R. Taylor et al. (1985). Comparison of ivermectin and diethylcarbamazine in the treatment of onchocerciasis. *New England Journal of Medicine* 313: 133–138

Greenhalgh, T. (2001). *How to Read a Paper: The Basics of Evidence Based Medicine*. London, BMJ Books

Grunbaum, A. (1981). The placebo concept. *Behavioral Research and Therapy* 19: 157–167

Haggard, H.W. (1934). *The Doctor in History*. New Haven, Yale University Press

Hamilton, G. (2001). Dead man walking. *New Scientist* 171(2303): 30

Hashish, I., H.K. Hai et al. (1988). Reduction of postoperative pain and swelling by ultrasound treatment: a placebo effect. *Pain* 33: 303–311

Hashish, I., W. Harvey et al. (1986). Anti-inflammatory effects of ultrasound therapy: evidence for a major placebo effect. *British Journal of Rheumatology* 25: 77–81

Hay, L.L. (1984). *You Can Heal Your Life*. Enfield, Eden Grove Editions

Healey, D. (1997). *The Antidepressant Era*. Cambridge, MA and London, Harvard University Press

Herrnstein, R.J. (1962). Placebo effect in the rat, *Science* 138: 677–678

Hill, A.B. (1963). Medical ethics and controlled trials. *British Medical Journal* 1: 1043–1049

Holroyd, K.A. and D.B. Penzian (1990). Pharmacological versus non-pharmacological prophylaxis of recurrent migraine headache: a meta-analytic review of clinical trials. *Pain* 42: 1–13

House of Lords Select Committee on Science and Technology (2000). Complementary and Alternative Medicine (HL Paper 123). London, Stationery Office

Hrobjartsson, A. and P.C. Gotzsche (2001). Is the placebo powerless? An analysis of clinical trials comparing placebo with no treatment. *New England Journal of Medicine* 344: 1594–1602

Humphrey, N. (2000). Great expectations: the evolutionary psychology of faith-healing and the placebo effect. *The Mind Made Flesh: Essays from the Frontier of Evolution and Psychology*. N. Humphrey. Oxford, Oxford University Press, 2002: 255–285

Ingelfinger, F.J. (1980). Arrogance. *New England Journal of Medicine* 303: 1507–11

Kaptchuk, T.J., R.A. Edwards et al. (1996). Complementary medicine: efficacy beyond the placebo effect. *Complementary Medicine: An Objective Appraisal*. Ed. E. Ernst. Oxford, Butterworth-Heinemann: 42–70

Kennedy, W.P. (1961). The nocebo reaction. *Medical World* 91: 203–205

Kent, S., R.-M. Bluthe et al. (1992). Sickness behaviour as a new target for drug development. *Trends in Pharmacological Sciences* 13: 24–28

Kienle, G.S. and H. Kiene (1997). The powerful placebo effect: fact or fiction? *Journal of Clinical Epidemiology* 50(12): 1311–1318

Kirsch, I. and G. Sapirstein (1998). Listening to Prozac but hearing placebo: a meta-analysis of antidepressant medication. *Prevention and Treatment* 1, Article 0002a. http://journals.apa.org/prevention/volume1/pre0010002a.html

Kirschbaum, C., I. Jabaij et al. (1992). Conditioning of drug-induced immunomodulation in human volunteers: a European collaborative study. *British Journal of Clinical Psychology* 31: 459–472

Klein, D.F. (1998). Listening to meta-analysis but hearing bias. *Prevention and Treatment* 1: Article 0006c. http://www.journals.apa.org/prevention/volume1/pre0010006c.html

Kleinman, A. (1988). *Rethinking Psychiatry*. New York, Free Press

Klopfer, B. (1957). Psychological variables in human cancer. *Journal of Projective Techniques* 21: 221–340

Kluger, M.J. (1979). *Fever: Its Biology, Evolution and Function.* Princeton, Princeton University Press

Kluger, M.J., W. Kozak et al. (2001). Fever and immunity. *Psychoneuroimmunology.* Eds R. Ader, D.L. Felten and N. Cohen. San Diego, Academic Press. 1: 687–701

Kruger, L., L.J. Daston et al., eds. (1987). *The Probabilistic Revolution. Volume I: Ideas in History.* Cambridge, MA and London, MIT Press

Lasagna, L. (1955). Placebos. *Scientific American* 193: 68–71

Launso, L. (1994). How to kiss a monster. *Studies in Alternative Therapy* 1. Eds H. Johannessen, L. Launso, S. Gosvigolesen and F. Stangard. Denmark, Odense University Press

Le Fanu, J. (1999). *The Rise and Fall of Modern Medicine.* London, Little, Brown

Lehmann, H.E. (1993). Before they called it psychopharmacology. *Neuropsychopharmacology* 8: 291–303

Levine, J.D., N.C. Gordon et al. (1978). The mechanism of placebo analgesia. *Lancet* 2: 654–657

Levi-Strauss, C. (1968). *Structural Anthropology,* Volume 1. Harmondsworth, Penguin

Lick, J.R. (1975). Expectancy, false galvanic skin response feedback and systematic desensitisation in the modification of phobic behaviour. *Journal of Counselling and Clinical Psychology* 43: 557–567

Lilienfeld, A.M. (1982). Ceteris paribus: the evolution of the clinical trial. *Bulletin of the History of Medicine* 56: 1–18

Linde, K., N. Clausius et al. (1997). Are the clinical effects of homeopathy placebo effects? A meta-analysis of placebo-controlled trials. *Lancet* 350: 834–843

Longo, D.L., P.L. Duffey et al. (1999). Conditioned immune response to interferon gamma in humans. *Clinical Immunology* 90(2): 173–81

Lynn, B. (1988). Neurogenic inflammation. *Skin Pharmacology* 1: 217–224

McQuay, H., D. Carroll et al. (1995). Variation in the placebo effect in randomised controlled trials of analgesics: all is as blind as it seems. *Pain* 64: 331–335

Maddox, J., J. Randi et al. (1988). 'High dilution' experiments a delusion. *Nature* 334: 287–290

Maes, M., E. Bosmans et al. (1991). Depression-related disturbances in mitogen-induced lymphocyte responses, interleukin–1B and soluble interleukin–2-receptor production. *Acta Psychiatrica Scandinavia* 84: 379–386

Maier, S.F., L.R. Waktins et al. (2001). Multiple routes of action of interleukin–1 on the nervous system. *Psychoneuroimmunology.* Eds R. Ader, D.L. Felten and N. Cohen. San Diego, Academic Press. 1: 563–583

Maier, S.F. and L.R. Watkins (1998). Cytokines for psychologists: implications of bidirectional immune-to-brain communication for understanding behavior, mood, and cognition. *Psychological Review* 105(1): 83–107

Martin, P. (1997). *The Sickening Mind: Brain, Behaviour, Immunity and Disease*. London, HarperCollins

Moerman, D.E. (2000). Cultural variations in the placebo effect: ulcers, anxiety, and blood pressure. *Medical Anthropology Quarterly* 14: 1–22

Montgomery, G.H. and I. Kirsch (1997). Classical conditioning and the placebo effect. *Pain* 72: 107–113

Morgan, E. (1990). *The Scars of Evolution*. Harmondsworth, Penguin

Moseley, J.B., N.P. Wray et al. (1996). Arthroscopic treatment of osteoarthritis of the knee: a prospective, randomized, placebo-controlled trial. Results of a pilot study. *American Journal of Sports Medicine* 24(1): 28–34

Motluk, A. (1999). Hearts and minds: treating depression can pave the way to a healthier heart. *New Scientist* 22 May 1999: 16

Nesse, R.M. and G. Williams (1994). *Why We Get Sick*. New York, Times Books

Nesse, R.M. (2000). Is depression an adaptation? *Archives of General Psychiatry* 57: 14–20

Park, I.C. and L. Covi (1965). Nonblind placebo trial. *Archives of General Psychiatry* 12: 336–345

Patel, M.S. (1987). Problems in the evaluation of alternative medicine. *Social Science Medicine* 25: 669–678

Pepper, O.H.P. (1945). A note on placebo. *Annual Journal of Pharmacology 2* 117: 409–12

Phillips, D.P. and D.G. Smith (1990). Postponement of death until symbolically meaningful occasions. *Journal of the American Medical Association* 263(14): 1947–51

Porter, R. (1997). *The Greatest Benefit to Mankind: A Medical History of Humanity from Antiquity to the Present*. London, HarperCollins

Prioleau, L., M. Murdock et al. (1983). An analysis of psychotherapy versus placebo studies. *Behavioral and Brain Sciences* 6: 275–285

Putsep, K., C.-I. Branden et al. (1999). Antibacterial peptide from H. pylori. *Nature* 398: 671–672

Rabkin, J.G., J.S. Markowitz et al. (1986). How blind is blind? Assessment of patient and doctor medication guesses in a placebo-controlled trial of imipramine and phenelzine. *Psychiatric Research* 19: 75–86

Randi, J. (1989). *The Faith Healers*. Amherst, NY, Prometheus Books

Rosenzweig, P., S. Brohier et al. (1993). The placebo effect in healthy volunteers: influence of experimental conditions on the adverse events profile during phase I studies. *Clinical Pharmacology and Therapeutics* 54(5): 578–583

Russell, B. (1971). *Logic and Knowledge*. New York, Putnam

Sackett, D.L., W.M.C. Rosenberg et al. (1996). Evidence based medicine: what it is and what it isn't. *British Medical Journal* 312: 71–2

Samal, S. and K.E. Geckeler (2001). Unexpected solute aggregation in water on dilution. *Chemical Communications* 21: 2224–2225

Sapolsky, R.M., S.C. Alberts et al. (1997). Hypercortisolism associated with social subordination or social isolation among wild baboons. *Archives of General Psychiatry* 54(12): 1137–1143

Schapira, K., H.A. McClelland et al. (1970). Study on the effects of tablet colour in the treatment of anxiety states. *British Medical Journal* 2: 446–449

Schmitt, B.D. (1980). Fever phobia: misconceptions of parents about fever. *American Journal of Diseases of Children* 134: 176–181

Segal, B. (1986). *Love, Medicine and Miracles.* New York, Harper & Row

Senn, S. (2001). The misunderstood placebo. *Applied Clinical Trials* 10: 40–46

Shapiro, A.K. (1960). A contribution to a history of the placebo effect. *Behavioural Science* 5: 109–35

Shapiro, A.K. and E. Shapiro (1997a). The placebo: is it much ado about nothing? *The Placebo Effect: An Interdisciplinary Exploration.* Ed. A. Harrington. Cambridge, MA and London, Harvard University Press: 12–36

Shapiro, A.K. and E. Shapiro (1997b). *The Powerful Placebo: From Ancient Priest to Modern Physician.* Baltimore and London, Johns Hopkins University Press

Shapiro, S. (1994). Meta-analysis, shmeta-analysis. *American Journal of Epidemiology* 140(9): 771–778

Smith, G.R. and S.M. McDaniels (1983). Psychologically mediated effect on the delayed hypersensitivity reaction to tuberculin. *Psychosomatic Medicine* 45: 65–68

Smith, M.L., G.V. Glass et al. (1980). *The Benefits of Psychotherapy.* Baltimore, Johns Hopkins University Press

Smith, M.L. and G.V. Glass (1977). Meta-analysis of psychotherapy outcome studies. *American Psychologist* 32: 752–760

Spiegel, D. (1997). Psychosocial aspects of breast cancer treatment. *Seminars in Oncology* 24((S1)): 36

Spiegel, D., J.R. Bloom et al. (1989). Effect of psychosocial treatment on survival of patients with metastatic breast cancer. *Lancet* 2(8668): 888–91

Spiro, H. (1997). Clinical reflections on the placebo phenomenon. *The Placebo Effect: An Interdisciplinary Exploration.* Ed. A. Harrington. Cambridge, MA and London, Harvard University Press: 37–55

Stein, D.M. and M.J. Lambert (1984). On the relationship between therapist experiences and psychotherapy outcomes. *Clinical Psychology Review* 4: 1–16

Stradling, J.R. and R.J.O. Davies (1997). The unacceptable face of evidence based medicine. *Journal for the Evaluation of Clinical Practice* 3: 99–103

Strupp, H. and S. Hadley (1979). Specific versus nonspecific factors in psychotherapy. *Archives of General Psychiatry* 36: 1125–1136

Svensson, E., L. Raberg et al. (1998). Energetic stress, immunosuppression and the costs of an antibody response. *Functional Ecology* 12: 912–19

Talbot, M. (2000). The placebo prescription. *New York Times Magazine*, 1 September 2000

Taylor, T. (1996). *The Prehistory of Sex: Four Million Years of Human Sexual Culture*. London, Bantam Books

Vickers, A. (1996). Research paradigms in mainstream and complementary medicine. *Complementary Medicine: An Objective Appraisal*. Ed. E. Ernst. Oxford, Butterworth-Heinemann: 1–17

Voudouris, N.J., C.L. Peck et al. (1989). Conditioned response models of placebo phenomena: further support. *Pain* 38: 109–116

Wall, P.D. (1999a). The placebo and the placebo response. *Textbook of Pain*, Fourth Edition. Ed. P.D. Wall. Edinburgh, Churchill: 1419–1430

Wall, P.D (1999b). *Pain: The Science of Suffering*. London, Weidenfeld & Nicolson

Watkins, A. and G. Lewith (1997). Mind-body medicine: its popularity and perception. *Mind-Body Medicine: A Clinician's Guide to Psychoneuroimmunology*. Ed. A. Watkins. New York, Churchill Livingston: 27–40

Weil, A. (1995). *Spontaneous Healing*. London, Little, Brown

Wickramasekera, I. (1980). A conditioned response model of the placebo effect: predictions from the model. *Biofeedback and Self-Regulation* 5: 5–18

Wolff, H.G., E.F. DuBois et al. (1946). Cornell conferences on therapy: use of placebos in therapy. *New York Journal of Medicine* 46: 1718–27

Wolpert, L. and D. Evans (2001). Malignant sadness: the evolutionary psychology of depression. Every Family in the Land. A.H. Crisp, http://www.stigma.org/everyfamily/

INDEX

acetaminophen 132
acupuncture xv, 141: clinical trials
   145–6, 148; patient contact 159;
   placebo effect and 70, 144–6, 153,
   155, 157, 159, 173; risks 142;
   theory of 144, 162
acute phase protein 52
acute phase response 44–69:
   activation of 44–58, 124, 128, 140,
   203; evolution of 98, 138–40;
   placebo-responsive conditions and
   44, 51–6, 63–70, 124, 134–5, 191;
   stages in process 45–51, 60–1, 68;
   suppression of 62–72, 98, 113–14,
   124, 127, 128, 134–5, 191, 202,
   203; see also inflammation
Ader, Robert 100–1
Adler, Alfred 166, 174–5
adrenal gland 51, 139
adrenaline 90–1
adrenocorticotropic hormone
   (ACTH) 51
alcohol 4, 164, 165
alternative and complementary
   medicine 141–63: beliefs 141–2,
   146–7, 158, 162, 173, 203;
   consumer satisfaction 154, 155,
   157; ethics of 162–3, 180, 181–91,
   196–8; evidence for 142–5;
   physical contact with clients
   159–60, 161; placebo effect and
   xv, 13, 143–6, 153–7, 160, 161–3,

180–3, 191, 196–8, 200; popularity
   xiii, 17, 142–3, 157; research on
   143–54; rift with orthodox
   medicine 133, 141–2, 146–7,
   151–2, 154–5, 157, 161, 162; risks
   of 142; ritual 158, 161; side-effects
   142; spending on 142; time given
   to clients 157–8, 161; see also types
   of therapies
Alzheimer's disease 64, 188
American Academy of Paediatrics 132
American Handbook of Psychiatry 166–7
American Medical Association 19
American Psychologist 167
analgesia 1, 2, 28–33, 46, 132:
   placebo 28–34, 52–3, 56–8, 81,
   113–14, 153, 156, 191, 201
anecdotal evidence 20–3
angina 4, 12, 32–3, 67–9
animals, non-human: beliefs and
   77–8; conditioning and 81–2, 86,
   100, 176; immune systems 137–40;
   placebo response and 99–101
antibiotic 135, 183
antibody 103
antidepressant 38–41, 69
antipyretic 49, 67, 127, 134
antiseptic 8
anxiety: benefits of 137; heart disease
   and 68–9; immune response and
   44, 48, 52, 54–6, 69; placebo
   response and 4, 5, 27, 36–7, 41–3,

216